CATHERINE SHANAHAN, MD

Food
Rules

A Doctor's Guide to Healthy Eating

Big Box Books
Bedford, NH

Every effort has been made to ensure that the information contained in the book is complete and accurate. However, neither the author nor the publisher is engaged in rendering advice to the individual reader.

Food Rules
A Doctor's Guide to Healthy Eating

Copyright © 2010 by Catherine Shanahan, MD

Library of Congress Cataloging-in-Publication Data

Shanahan, Catherine MD
Food Rules: A Doctor's Guide to Healthy Living
Catherine Shanahan, MD

Library of Congress Control Number: 2010910126

Printed in the United States of America

To order, visit www.DrCate.com or Amazon.com
ISBN-13: 9-781452-861388

To everyone who is kind to animals.

Contents

Introduction

Part One: What should I buy?
(Buy natural)

Part Two: How Should I Cook?
(According to tradition)

Part Three: How should I eat? (Eat Mindfully)

Doctor's Orders

Appendices

Is Your Problem Inflammation?

If you have taken steps to be healthy but your diet and/or exercise program hasn't produced the results you want, there is a good chance the reason is inflammation. Most of the health problems that bring people into my office stem from inflammation caused by dietary imbalance. Once your body is trapped in an inflammatory cycle, you can no longer eliminate fat cells or transform them into muscle. Inflammation is the wall that stands between you and the body you want. *If you want to get healthy and lose weight, you first need to tear down that wall.*

To appreciate how inflammation can promote weight gain and other chronic diseases you have to know something about the role of inflammation in your body.

In a healthy body, inflammation serves a useful purpose. When you sprain your ankle, for instance, torn tissues trigger a cascade of inflammatory responses that increase blood flow and cause visible swelling. Beneath the distended skin lies a demolition zone where inflammatory reactions are clearing out damaged parts to make room for repairs that will ultimately rebuild your ankle joint. When you catch a cold, viruses in your lymph nodes trigger inflammation that gets them started making antibodies, and a sore throat and stuffy nose are symptoms of the battle in your oral and upper airway passages. Normally, once the ankle sprain or cold has resolved, the inflammation subsides.

In the setting of dietary imbalance, however, inflammation takes longer to go away—much longer. Because inflammation blocks normal metabolic function and disturbs cellular growth, not only will minor injuries and infections take longer to clear, serious diseases like atherosclerosis and cancer are likely to develop.

1

The word inflammation comes from the Latin *inflammare*, "to set on fire," and the sensations it causes will depend on where the "fire" smolders. If you have inflammation in your joints, you feel aching and stiffness. In your gut, nausea and cramping. In your head, a headache. In the lungs, it can make you cough. Inflammation can also cause tiredness, irritability, hormonal problems, allergies, and more. These common symptoms are often attributed to age, stress, infections, or carrying extra weight, but all should be taken as warning signs that your diet is harming your body.

Inflammation also prevents your body from building muscle, which limits your ability to see weight loss and muscle gain from exercise. Since fat cells can exude inflammatory chemicals, excessive fat (i.e., a BMI over 25) acts as an inflammation-generating machine and may trap you in a vicious cycle of weight gain, inflammation, and still more weight gain. Attempting to reverse this cycle simply by eating fewer of the same pro-inflammatory foods may produce temporary results but, since it does little to address inflammation, typically fails over the long term.

What you need is a metabolic makeover. If you are suffering from any illness listed below, the rules in this book will help you, first by clearing your body of inflammation and then by giving you the foods you need to regenerate healthy new tissues.

<u>Inflammation Causes or Worsens Many Diseases, Including:</u>

- Overweight
- Diabetes/prediabetes
- Cancer
- Allergies and asthma
- Anxiety
- Headaches
- Learning disorders

- Neuropathy
- Fatty liver and heartburn
- Arthritis and tendonitis
- Atherosclerosis
- Hypertension
- Polycystic ovaries
- Chronic fatigue

Why I Focus on Diet

How often do you turn on the TV and see a story about a child affected by autism, a mother with breast cancer, the lack of effective Alzheimer's treatments, or the obesity epidemic? It's not just media hype. The CDC has predicted that the generation of children born in 2000 will be the first in recorded history to have a shorter lifespan than their parents, while skyrocketing healthcare costs have been identified as a potential threat to our national security. If our accelerating health crises have any single underlying cause, I believe it may be this: *Doctor's don't study nutrition.*

Medical school is notorious for underemphasizing nutrition. Doctors do not learn enough about the way in which harmful inflammation and degeneration combine to cause the diseases most of their patients experience. Unless we've studied independently, we physicians can't offer many insights into how our patients' food choices contributed to the problems that brought them in. Nor do we offer sound advice on what to eat or how to cook to stay out of a hospital. While doctors are well aware of the potential for a profound connection between diet and health, we become convinced through our training that we shouldn't bother talking to our patients about the food they put into their bodies unless they are overweight. Even then, conversations are extremely superficial and usually go something like this:

MD: *Are you watching what you eat?*

Patient: *Well, doc, I'm trying to, but I usually just watch it all go right into my mouth!*

MD: *Ha, ha. Well, try to moderate your intake a little bit.*

In years past, I too was guilty of glossing over the topic with my patients. Before doing any research related to my first book,

Deep Nutrition, I only talked about diet with people who were severely overweight or diabetic, and limited those discussions to what little I knew: *Count your calories. Try to exercise. Chose low-fat.* That was the extent of my advice because I assumed that was all one needed to know. I'd figured my curriculum had largely omitted the subject of nutrition because nutrition didn't really matter. I also assumed that family history and genes had more to do with my patients' health than their diets; I had no idea that food can change the course of a family's health by influencing genetic expression. I underestimated the power of nutrition to hurt or heal. And so, like most doctors, I focused on medications.

If you are eating the kinds of foods most of my patients are eating when they first come to see me, the bulk of your caloric intake is made of grain and legume starches and sugars, fruit sugars, low-quality meats from animals also fed grains and legumes (as opposed to grass and other forage), and vegetable oils—exactly what the government tells you to eat. Contrast this monotony against what our great-great-grandparents ate a hundred years ago: bone broths, organ meats, fermented fruits and vegetables, fresh (unpasteurized) butter and naturally soured dairy. This migration away from real food to edible industrial products tells us all we need to know about the cause of our sickness epidemic.

Because most health professionals are oblivious to the lost variety in our diets, as a group we are simply unqualified to provide nutritional advice. Worse, the American economy is now dependent on big pharma and other industries that sell services to sick people for more than thirty percent of our GDP. In other words, if nobody is sick, that's bad for thirty percent of American industry. Where is the incentive to look for real solutions?

This has created a vacuum in the business of healthcare. Patients now rely on alternative practitioners to provide what their own physicians cannot. Many of these alternative providers are among our nation's most informed and progressive thinkers in the science of human health. Others, however, are as ill equipped to defend their dietary recommendations as are most physicians. Lacking a central clearinghouse—a formalized peer review system—in which competing nutritional theories can be tested, patients are left confused over what are often conflicting and incompatible philosophies.

With my background in biochemistry and genetics, and clinical experience with the effects of a variety of dietary programs, I have successfully guided thousands of patients through this shifting landscape of competing ideologies. This book represents the core of my nutritional advice, a simple, easy-to-follow set of rules that will produce the results you've been looking for.

The Anti-Inflammation Diet

The rules in this book are based in the science explained in detail in *Deep Nutrition* and represent the key elements of T.R.I.M. (Treatment to Reverse Inflammatory Metabolism), my successful weight-loss program. During initial consultation with patients, I have noticed many questions coming up again and again. So before we dive into the rules, I thought it might be good to address some of the most common right up front.

What kind of diet is this?

This is your guide to reproducing the kind of diet the healthiest people followed generations ago, before the invention of industrial food. You can apply these rules to make any dish in the world, to enjoy an unlimited variety of authentic cuisines that will regenerate your health by reducing the inflammation that interferes with your metabolic balance and genetic expression.

Is this diet low-carb?

Yes. All carbs—even whole grains—raise blood sugar. A few decades of carb-centered eating (making bread, rice, pasta, etc. a part of every meal) damages your metabolism so that you feel energy lows and hunger pangs that make you want to eat more than you need. As you will learn, more than 100-150 grams of carbohydrate per day lead to inflammation and weight gain, while diets high in natural fat are anti-inflammatory.

Won't fat make me fat?

Natural fats don't make us fat. Trans fat, particularly in combination with sugar, practically guarantees weight gain. A deficiency of (natural) fat in your diet makes it difficult for you to burn fat. And you can't lose weight without burning fat.

Why don't you worry about fat raising my cholesterol?

The cholesterol number that matters is your HDL to LDL ratio, not your total cholesterol. Because inflammation breaks down cholesterol-carrying particles in ways that can damage your arteries, we've been mislead into thinking cholesterol is the cause of the problem when it is not. Low HDL and high triglyceride numbers are better indicators of your risk of heart attack and stroke than LDL or total cholesterol.

I eat my vegetables, isn't that good enough?

Not really. Have you had liver in the past week? What about soup or gravy made from bone broth? Or sauerkraut/pickles/kimchee containing probiotic (good) bacteria? Two hundred years ago, you would probably have said yes to all three, but today most Americans can go decades without even seeing them. Your great-grandparents' survival depended on these foods, and if you want medication independence, so does yours.

Why doesn't my doctor know about this?

Here's a little story that may help answer that question. Back in 2004, Boston University's Dr. Michael Holick publicized the fact that up to eighty percent of Americans are deficient in vitamin D, which may double their risk of colon, breast, and prostate cancer. Then, Holick suggested holding the sunscreen occasionally in favor of sensible UV exposure. That single recommendation was radical enough to get him fired from his post as Chair of the Dermatology department. This is the kind of political backlash that prevents most academics from rocking the boat. Only after he published a book that explained his reasoning, and only after alternative practitioners started prescribing vitamin D, did the medical establishment pick up on the story, sometime in 2009. This tells you something about the difficulties medical leaders encounter when they actually try to lead.

How did you learn about inflammation?

Before medical school I studied biochemistry and molecular biology at Cornell University where I learned how nature operates inside living cells. During my years of medical practice, I came to appreciate that disrupting the natural order of cellular function causes disease. Thanks to this combination of education in the basic sciences and clinical experience I can now explain which foods and processing steps promote inflammation. For example, I now warn people that processing milk with pasteurization and homogenization leads to more allergies than consuming it fresh, that overcooking otherwise healthy salmon destroys omega-3 fatty acids, and that canola oils contain a kind of trans fat that can damage cells and DNA. The T.R.I.M. philosophy rests on the understanding that eliminating inflammation enables your body to naturally restore metabolic balance.

Can this little book really tell me all I need to know?

Learning to take command of your health is a lifelong journey. But many people want a simple, concise, foolproof guide to get them started in the right direction. This book is that guide. For a more complete understanding of how these dietary changes will affect your body, your cells, and your genes, read *Deep Nutrition*.

But I heard (blank) was good/bad for me...

When patients ask about the health benefits or harms of particular foods, often dairy, grains, soy, or meat, I help them answer the question for themselves by going back to source and tradition. If *any* food comes from the same kind of source as people who traditionally relied on it, and was prepared in the same manner, it's likely going to be good for you. If either source or preparation has changed, then you are not going to get the same benefits.

How are these rules arranged?

Part One will help you shop healthy. You'll learn what to buy, which kinds of markets and stores to patronize, when to shop organic, and how to decide between two brands of the same thing.

Part Two will help you to start thinking about food and nutrition like a chef. It's no accident that Julia Child lived to 91. Rather than limiting you to dependence on a few included recipes, I focus on tips and techniques to make it easier for you to choose the best recipes from what's freely available on the Web.

Part Three will help you curb overeating and guide you toward a healthier relationship with food.

Doctor's Orders provides must-know essentials to learn before your next visit to the doctor. It covers the best, most valuable lab tests and the worst, most over-prescribed prescription drugs.

Finally, what is your philosophy on health and healing?

Health is the inevitable result of obeying nature's rules and disease is the inevitable result of distancing your body from nature. I offer you these rules to help you make nature your ally. If you follow them closely, nature will reward you.

Part One: What should I buy? (Buy natural)

The first step in knowing what to buy is understanding the function of food. Food does far more than provide you with calories and a few vitamins and minerals. Food carries vital information that connects the cells of your body to a specific ecology in the soil or the sea. Put simply, food is nature you can eat.

The best foods remind us of their origins. Fresh fish smells like ocean; colorful, aromatic vegetables speak of rich, black soil, clean water, and sunshine; the deep orange-yellow egg yolk tells us good things about the diet of the hen that laid it, her living conditions, and even something about the farmer.

This section will help you avoid some of the most common shopping pitfalls (like trusting the words "All Natural" on the label) and provide you with some simple tips to help you best convert your money into units of consumable nature.

(1)
Buy natural.

Natural has become a meaningless term. Anyone who wants to use the word "natural" on their food label can because there is no specific legal requirement for doing so. Besides, you can make laser-jet ink out of soybeans, car fuel out of corn, and buttons out of milk protein—natural ingredients all, but you wouldn't want to eat them. The point is, you shouldn't buy anything simply because it has the word "natural" on the label or because something "healthy" has been added (think crackers with added fiber).

It's far easier to start by defining what is *not* natural. Most of us agree that when we talk about highly processed foods we've moved into the realm of the unnatural. Now the question becomes *How do we identify those foods that are highly processed?* Here's where the label can work for us. Processed foods are easily identified by any of these three ingredients: Vegetable oil, sugar, and MSG. Either ingredient appearing alone is cause for alarm. If all three show up together on the same label, then you can be sure you are looking at a highly processed, very unnatural, and very unhealthy food product. Put it down and back away slowly.

(2)
Avoid vegetable oils.

Avoiding vegetable oils requires some skill, but it is perhaps the most important shopping skill for you to master.

Most people now know that hydrogenated oils contain large quantities of trans fat and other toxic fats. Few people know that vegetable oils are processed in a similar series of steps. The toxic chemicals in vegetable oils and hydrogenated oils damage cells and disrupt basic metabolic function, and have been linked to serious health problems, including genetic damage, birth defects, growth anomalies, cancer, heart attacks, strokes, and more. I let my patients know that if they make vegetable oils part of their diet, it's not a question of when the stuff will make them sick, it's only a question of how.

Avoid these oils:

- Canola oil
- Corn oil
- Soy oil
- Cottonseed oil
- Sunflower oil
- Safflower oil
- Grapeseed oil
- Rice bran oil

Don't panic when you discover the extent to which these food-industry novelties have seeped into our food supply. Although, in terms of raw calories, they now represent at least a third of most people's daily intake, there are better, tastier alternatives. Once you've managed to turn the vegetable oil spigot off, your health will begin to improve immediately.

Avoid these foods if they contain any vegetable oil:

- Chocolates (look for cocoa butter or milk fat. Dove, Hershey's, and most organic chocolates use healthier fats)
- Salad dressings (dressings are super easy to make anyway, see Rules)
- Cookies (look for butter)
- Granola (look for coconut or olive oil)
- Breakfast cereal (this eliminates most boxed cereals, see the breakfast menu in the appendices)
- Bread (most commonly used vegetable oils for bread making are canola and soy. Look for breads made with healthier oils or no oil)

What makes vegetable oils so nasty?

During factory refining, all vegetable oils are superheated (including "expeller pressed"). Vegetable oils contain polyunsaturated fats that are damaged by heat. And so, all vegetable oils contain a variety of incredibly harmful molecules, most notoriously *trans* fats, but there are many others. In Canada, consumers can find the trans fatty acid content right on the bottle's label. Unfortunately, in America, oil bottles do not warn us, and few people have any idea of the hazards incurred by consuming these benign-sounding ingredients.

(3)
Buy healthy oils.

Healthy oils are those that, with a wedge or stone press (and some motivation), you could produce in your own home. These are the oils that have been used for generations. Unlike vegetable oils, these wonderful oils are more like foods—the best examples are fresh, aromatic, unrefined (often cloudy), and swimming with healthy phytochemicals.

These are the oils you should buy:

- Olive
- Peanut
- Coconut
- Cocoa butter
- Avocado
- Macadamia nut
- Sesame
- Walnut
- Flax seed
- Wheat germ oil

We'll talk about which of these oils are suitable for cooking with in a later rule.

(4)
Kick your sugar addiction.

Sugar is an addictive drug. I mean that literally. Sugar consumption releases *endogenous opiates*, brain chemicals that make you feel so good that you do things you know are stupid just to get that feeling again. I once drove 200 miles across the state of North Dakota for a Mocha-Frappuccino to learn, after stepping up to the counter, that they'd just run out.

The side effects of sugar consumption include, but are not limited to, reduced immune function, increased fat production, fatty liver, heart palpitations, hypertension, anxiety, and diabetes. Add vegetable oil to your sugary diet and all of these unhealthy side effects are magnified.

If you are not sure whether you are a sugar addict or not, here's a test: If sweets regularly give you that euphoric, roll-your-eyes-back, don't-you-dare-take-this-from-me, mmmm-good-feeling, you're addicted. Take it from a former sugarholic, once you kick the habit and cut way back on sugar, everything tastes better and you will experience your favorite foods—from cheese to chocolate—in a whole new way.

(5)
Don't be fooled: sugar is sugar.

Since many health-conscious consumers are on the lookout for sugar, food manufacturers have responded by hiding it every way they can. They change the name (fructose, maltose, dextrose—see list), or tell us it's actually "healthy sugar" (honey, agave nectar, fruit sugar), or, if all else fails, they add a low-calorie artificial sweetener.

Sugar is sugar and it's always bad for you.

Learn to recognize some common sugar pseudonyms:

- Evaporated cane juice
- Corn syrup
- Corn sweeteners
- High fructose corn syrup
- Fructose
- Sucrose
- Malt
- Malt syrup
- Barley malt syrup
- Barley malt extract
- Maltose
- Maltodextrin
- Brown rice syrup
- Maple syrup
- Dextrose

- Beet juice
- Molasses
- Honey
- Grape juice (usually added to jellies and jams)
- Muscovado (partially refined molasses)
- Turbinado (more highly refined molasses)
- Sucanat (a version of brown sugar)
- Invert sugar
- Agave nectar
- Xylose

(6)
Treat carbs as sugar—*They are!*

To reduce your sugar intake you need to cut your carbs. Starches are composed of sugar molecules (mainly glucose); hold a cracker on your tongue for a full minute and it will begin to taste sweet as your saliva starts to break the starches down. Once fully digested, starches—whether complex or simple—enter your blood stream as sugar. So eliminate food bars, and keep all other carb sources including fruit to two or three total servings per day on average. If you have a bagel for breakfast an apple and a sandwich at lunch, for instance, then you should not routinely have rice, potatoes, or pasta for dinner.

Carbs are mostly empty calories, and the more serious you are about your health, the more seriously you need to stick to this rule. Limiting yourself to one or two servings of carbs per day will cut inflammation and get your metabolism into shape faster than three or four.

These foods can raise blood sugar:

- Pasta
- Bread
- Rice
- Potatoes
- Noodles

- Corn
- Breakfast cereals and bars
- "Health" and energy bars
- Crackers
- Fruit

Whole grains are better than refined, but they will raise your blood sugar much like their white-colored cousins and their benefits are overhyped. Brown rice is not much better than white: 89 percent starch versus 96, give or take, depending on the strains and how they were milled. All starch, whether from whole grains or refined, enters your bloodstream as sugar. Even quinoa and millet and the other "old world" cereal grains, along with corn—which is very starchy—are mostly starch and will raise blood sugar.

You can have pasta, mashed potatoes, bread, and other healthy starchy foods without guilt. But if you've been having more than two servings a day, it's time to replace some of that starch with other, more nutrient-dense foods (for instance, by putting more sauce on the pasta—*especially* if it's homemade).

If you are a healthy athlete with an ideal body weight, you are okay exceeding the two-serving rule as long as you balance any extra carbs with a roughly equal amount of calories from fat.

It is a common misperception that certain cuisines are traditionally based on starch. Over the last few generations the price of seafood and vegetables has increased, sometimes dramatically, while the price of grains and starch has not kept pace. This financial reality has changed the character of the meals in many countries. Just because starch has suddenly become the world's most readily affordable food doesn't make it good for us.

Why is sugar so bad? Sugar is sticky and that stickiness affects your inner biology in a profound way. Sticky sugars bind to your body's moving parts, most painfully the collagen in your joints. Sugar also binds to the proteins in your cell membranes, aging them and literally shutting them down. I go into more detail on how sugar's stickiness makes it potentially toxic to your tissues in *Deep Nutrition*.

(7)

Don't buy artificial sweeteners.

Think of Splenda, Nutrasweet, and saccharine as sweet-tasting drugs. They create the taste you're after with fewer calories but not without side effects—everything from blurry vision to intestinal tumors to cancer.

On the other hand, stevia is a natural sweetener, kind of like a spice. It's expensive, but can be used to sweeten coffee and tea. I advise against ritual use of all sweeteners, however, based on the fact that they're habit forming and can take over your diet in an unhealthy way. If you use stevia to sweeten baked goods or ice cream in an effort to cut calories, forget it. Unless you also cut back on your portion sizes, you'll just be eating more of the other ingredients.

The sweetness receptors in your intestines—taste buds in your gut—react to all sweetness, whether from sugar, stevia, or artificial sources, the same way. This "gut perception" of sweetness initiates insulin production, which can, in turn, raise LDL levels and promote the production of fat.

Even if artificial sweeteners were relatively safe, like stevia, I'd still advise you to save your money for real food. These products desensitize your palate to the sweetness nature puts in almost everything.

(8)
Avoid foods containing MSG.

Just as there are good fats and bad, there are good proteins and bad. MSG is a bad one. MSG is named after its main component, the amino acid glutamate, which doesn't exist in natural food as it does in Mono Sodium Glutamate (MSG). It's not that glutamate is inherently unnatural; it's just that when consumed alone, as an isolated amino acid, it has potentially toxic effects.

Here's the good side of glutamate. Glutamate creates a potent taste sensation because it can bind directly to taste buds. Along with the four well-known taste sensations humans experience—sweet, salty, sour, bitter—glutamate adds a fifth, called *umami* (Japanese for "good flavor"). Umami satisfies our body's hunger for amino acids while providing our palates with the perception of deep, rich complexity. In traditional cuisines, the umami flavor derives naturally from roasting meats and vegetables, and from fermenting foods to make things like pickles, soy sauce, and miso, all of which contain glutamate in a natural form (as a peptide, not as a *lone* amino acid—hence the *mono* in MSG).

In mono sodium glutamate, the lone glutamate amino acid is bonded with sodium salt. Free glutamate triggers the very same taste sensors in the tongue as nourishing foods, tricking our brains into thinking we've found a complete protein source when we're actually getting only the one amino acid. Manufacturers who use MSG can entice us to eat stale nuts, overcooked, freezer-burned mystery meats, and way more starch than we need. Always remember, *If it says MSG, it's no good for me.*

(9)
Avoid free glutamate.

Not all manufacturers want to make avoiding MSG so simple. So how do they slip it by the health-conscious shopper? Most often, as a protein powder or slurry. Look for HSP (hydrolyzed soy protein) or HVP (hydrolyzed vegetable protein), two of the most common names for protein powders with MSG-like effects on your taste buds.

Food makers have good reason to hide the fact that their products contain MSG. They know that many consumers want to avoid MSG because it causes headaches. MSG has been linked to a variety of other nervous system disorders, including temporary memory loss and aphasia (an inability to talk). Because the glutamate in MSG can cross the blood-brain barrier and overstimulate nerves to the point of malfunction, it has been dubbed an "excitotoxin." Weight-conscious consumers should be most concerned with the fact that this excitotoxic compound induces you to eat more than you should, detonating your diet plans the moment you tear into a new sack of chips (see also Rule 57).

(10)
Avoid foods containing MSG—
Especially if you're a vegetarian.

Have you ever had a steaming bowl of rice drizzled with Bragg's Liquid Aminos? Not only is it so delicious you just can't stop eating, it's supposed to be really good for you.

It isn't. Look on the label and you won't find MSG, and it doesn't contain MSG per se, but it's made by a process that is very similar to the MSG manufacturing process, called protein hydrolysis. Hydrolysis breaks the protein apart, releasing individual amino acids. In the case of soy protein, which is high in the amino acid glutamate, hydrolysis releases enough free glutamate to have MSG-like effects on the nervous system. When Bragg's—or anything containing free glutamate–is consumed without meat, these lone amino acids pass more readily across the blood-brain barrier, potentially manifesting excitotoxic damage.

(11)
Avoid foods containing MSG—
Especially with alcohol.

Alcohol weakens the blood-brain barrier and makes it much easier for free glutamate to get to your brain and damage nerves. This subset of the "Avoid free glutamate rule" deserves its own page because I have treated several patients who were hospitalized with stroke-like symptoms. All of them broke this rule (and none actually had strokes). Their symptoms resolved within 48 hours and, before I sent them home, I taught them how to identify hidden MSG.

Besides searching labels for protein powders and "hydrolysates," you should also look for anything containing "natural flavors." A consumer group found that 95 percent of such products contain MSG.

(12)
Want your umami.

As I've noted, umami is the fifth taste, and the Japanese word for "good flavor." The umami sensation is supposed to signal the presence of complex nutrients, so our craving for umami is a good thing. In fact, some of the healthiest foods and condiments you can buy are characterized by their umami flavor.

Get your umami from these healthy sources:

- Fermented pickles, sauerkraut, and kimchee
- Real, fermented tofu (if you can find it)
- Artisanal sausages and cured meats (made with "lactic acid starter culture" and without nitrates or nitrites)
- Raw milk cheeses
- Kikkoman and other authentic, naturally brewed soy sauces
- Fish sauce (as with soy sauces, the good brands will also say "naturally brewed" or "fermented")
- Oyster sauce (the best brands list oysters as a top ingredient; the cheap ones, water)

(13)
Don't buy foods that lie to you.

If you're serious about a healthy diet, you probably already know to avoid foods that pretend to be something they're not. Margarine, sugar substitutes, and soy milk are better left on the shelf until they resolve their identity crisis.

Some foods do more than play make-believe; they flat out lie to you on the label. Spreads and salad dressings claiming to be made with olive oil may contain only trace amounts. They'd rather sell you canola, or corn, or soy — or one of the other factory oils that cost much less. The fact that some food manufacturers pull this bait and switch should tell you something about the quality of their products.

(14)
Buy foods that vary in shape, color, and size whenever possible.

Restaurants, especially fast food chains, demand consistency in the ingredients they buy from their distributors so that they know how much to order and everything can be cooked exactly the same way. Consumers have gotten so accustomed to this lack of variation that they, too, demand that each potato, tomato, egg, and chicken breast appear identical to all others in the store. They also want them to look the same as they did last week—even if they were shopping on the opposite side of the country. This perfect consistency in food products is a hallmark of mass production and genetic cloning.

By contrast, variation in any food product is the hallmark of the local, independent farmer or fisherman and almost always says something good about the merchandise.

(15)
Pay more.

Consider what many of us have gone through to live in a better zip code, whether for a better school system, a safer neighborhood, or just the additional prestige. We may borrow well beyond our means under the assumption that a better neighborhood will improve the quality of our lives and the lives of our family.

We invest in real estate, but when it comes to food, many of us pinch pennies, effectively relegating our body's cells to the worst neighborhood in town. Every Thanksgiving, I hear people talking about where to buy the cheapest turkey. This infatuation with bargain hunting can come with a hefty price tag down the road. When considering free-range over feedlot, grass-fed over grain-fed, organic over industrial, also consider the cost to your health and the fact that a single admission to the hospital could easily wipe out a decade or two of those savings.

Calorie for calorie, real food does cost more money. It should; it costs more to produce. Feedlot beef from unhealthy cattle is far less nourishing than its grass-fed counterpart and is typically adulterated with tenderizers and petrochemicals. Pennies-per-pound-poultry comes from fowl whose legs buckle underneath their overgrown bulk, pumped-up further still with water and MSG. On the other hand, locally grown, organic vegetables typically contain several times more antioxidants than those shipped from thousands of miles away and ripened under a blanket of ethylene gas. Though it may seem expensive, in terms of nutrition per pollutant-free calorie, however, real food costs less.

27

Of course, it's easy for a doctor to tell you to pay more for better food. The hard part comes when you're a working mom or dad, or struggling student, roaming the aisles of a big box store where you can fill your cart for next to nothing. That's where you have to make a tough choice: Save your money, or save your health.

(16)
Shop for nutrition.

When we pay a lot of money for something, we tend to expect it to be really big—big cars, big houses, and big packages of food. This mentality can make it difficult to spend ten dollars on something really healthy, like a tin of salmon roe, when for the same money you can get a ten-pound sack of potatoes.

Think of it this way: Instead of shopping for food in terms of bulk, shop for the nutrition that's in the food. Although the salmon roe may not load down your cart the way the potatoes do, it represents far more nutrition. The potatoes are little more than empty calories and petrochemical residue.

If that trick doesn't work, see if this helps you to more effectively shop for nutrition: Imagine you'll have to carry all those groceries up and down stairs, load them in and out of your car, and stuff them into a pair of jeans—because that's what you'll be doing.

(17)
Always read ingredients.

My husband once brought home a package of dried blueberries that, it turned out, contained vegetable oil. I asked him to bring it back.

(18)
Make smart deli decisions

Cold cuts should look like meat, with real muscle fibers that fall apart like real meat, not a meat-sponge fusion. Take sliced chicken breast. The flesh should be the color and consistency of actual white meat and not have that rubbery, bologna consistency. Same goes for turkey. Skip bologna all together, or anything bologna-like. All spongy sandwich meat with that uniform pink color has been over-processed and preserved with nitrates. Avoid these.

A good deli will offer pâtés. These can be super-foods when made with liver and healthy fat. When buying liver and organ meats, it is especially important to ask about the source of the animals (if they were pastured, humanely raised, etc.). If the grocer doesn't have a clue what farm his products came from, that's not a good sign.

Choose these deli meats:
- Roast beef
- Chicken breast
- Turkey breast
- Chorizo
- Prosciutto
- Head cheese (lots of collagen, omega-3 fats)
- Liverwurst
- Jagdwurst
- Salami

(19)
Buy more vegetables and fewer fruits.

I sometimes wish they put fresh vegetables on one side of the store and fresh fruits on the other. Veggies are a health food, fruits, a treat. The familiar phrase "eat your fruits and vegetables" suggests the two are nutritionally equivalent. Hardly. Every doctor and diabetic who checks their blood sugar knows that fruit, like fruit juice, raises blood sugar levels. I'm not saying fruit is outright bad for you, just that calorie for calorie, vegetables deliver far more nutrients than sugar-laden fruits.

The fruits we're familiar with owe their current form to their ability to provide our taste buds with a massive amount of sugar. That's how we've bred them. The wild ancestors of today's apples, berries, melons, and other domesticated fruits bore little resemblance to their modern counterparts. Moreover, their seasons were fleeting and so access was limited. Along these lines, tart tasting fruits are going to be more nutritious than sweet ones: Red delicious apples are mostly sugar; Blueberries are a little better, more antioxidants, for instance; Cranberries—now we're getting somewhere; this tart fruit is bursting with flavor and phytonutrients.

Your vegetable-to-fruit purchase ratio should be five to one. Veggies, including things like tomatoes and peppers (technically fruits but we consider them "greens") may also contain some sugar, but if they don't taste sweet, it's not enough sugar to worry about.

Unless you're fermenting them, fruits and veggies are best for you when they're as freshly picked as possible.

Buy fresh vegetables, not frozen or canned.

If you feed kids freezer-burned broccoli, or a thawed-out block of frozen spinach, or peas and carrots that you bought last July, you may make them veggie-haters for life. Canning damages most nutrients, obliterating the B vitamins, and freezing takes its toll on antioxidants, like vitamin C and phytonutrients. These nutrients don't disappear. They fuse together to form useless, sometimes harmful compounds, and all these changes are reflected in those canned and frozen flavors. Get the fresh stuff.

(21)

Don't buy your kids sugary foods.

Some parental behavior baffles me. Lobbying for phthalate-free toys and plastic gadgets while buying kids sugary junk makes no sense. Phthalates interfere with sexual development. Sugar interferes with intellectual development, disrupts hormones governing normal growth, and programs genes for early-onset diabetes.

Don't get these for your kids:

- Fruit juices
- Cookies
- Sugary fruits, i.e., raisins
- Peanut butter (sugar-free is okay)
- Jelly
- Sweetened cold or hot cereals
- Soda
- Sports drinks
- Ice cream

If you see these foods in your shopping cart, you are letting the food manufacturers (who consistently push the idea that kids need sugar for energy) run your household.

I mean this literally. In my years of practice I have learned that when a parent comes in stressed out from out-of-control kids at home, it is a near certainty that the problems came from their shopping cart more than their parenting style. If every meal delivers an infusion of sugar, the child is caught in a turbulent cycle of energy highs followed by crushing fatigue when the buzz wears off. This is a recipe for household chaos—especially if you have more than one child. Switching your kids over to grown up food can be immediately transformative for their health, and *your* sanity.

(22)
Avoid (most) fruit juice.

I have never understood what's wrong with water, but I have had patients tell me they just can't stand the stuff. Wanting to be healthy, they buy fruit juice rather than soda. That's not much of an improvement.

Most fruit juices are sweetened. "100 percent pure orange juice," for instance, typically contains added corn syrup. Manufacturers can get away with this in secret because corn syrup contains the same fructose naturally present in the fruit, so the FDA doesn't consider it materially different from fruit juice and has not made it a requirement to reveal added corn syrup. Besides, there is no simple test that can tell if corn syrup has been added.

The fruit juices I recommend are the powerful-tasting kinds, like unsweetened cranberry or grapefruit. Those mouth-puckering flavors tell you that you are getting plenty of antioxidants and not too much sugar.

The fruit itself is better than its juice. A cup of grapefruit juice, for example, has 94 calories, almost no fiber, and no vitamin A. A cup of fresh grapefruit sections has 74 calories, 10 percent of the RDA of fiber, and 43 percent of the RDA of vitamin A.

Some of the healthiest fruit juices are made from wild fruits, such as acai and goji. Unfortunately, most of these exotic and expensive juices are reconstituted from dry powder and their antioxidant content has been drastically reduced. What's more, they can be so pungent that manufacturers add sugar—often in the form of fruit juices that have been doped with corn syrup.

(23)
Go to the store twice a week, minimum.

Shopping twice a week will keep you knee-deep in fresh greens. And produce, meats, and fish are typically delivered on different days of the week. To get the goods when they're at their peak, find out what comes in when. (There's so little fresh food in the aisles these days, you'll probably only have to track down one or two people per store.) In hot weather, bring a cooler with some of those reusable cold packs in your car.

(24)
Skip the skim.

Never buy skim or low-fat milk, yoghurt, or cheese. Full-fat dairy consumption has not been associated with weight gain, and studies show that people who drink whole milk and get more dairy fat in their diets live longer, have healthier bones, and are less likely to suffer from heart attacks. (For more details, see Archives of Pediatrics & Adolescent Medicine (2005) 159:543-550, and European Journal of Clinical Nutrition (2010) 64, 569 577.)

Pesticide and other chemical residues bioconcentrate in dairy fat, making it not so healthy. So if your budget only allows for a limited number of organic foods, spend those dollars on organic dairy.

(25)

Buy free-range eggs, especially if you're a vegetarian.

Eggs are one of nature's superfoods. To be really good for you, however, they have to come from healthy hens allowed access to sunlight (for vitamin D), natural forage (for vitamins A and K), and bugs (for omega-3 fatty acids). You can see the difference in the color of the yolk; free-range looks bright orange from all the nutrients, and grain-fed is a dull yellow. Just as I advise prioritizing your organic dollars for dairy, eggs should be at the top of your free-range list.

(26)
Buy raw milk and cheeses.

Let me tell you something you may never have heard: Raw milk and pasteurized, homogenized milk are completely different products. They may look similar, but at the microscopic level pasteurized, homogenized milk exposed to scalding heat and deforming pressure displays severe damage to its membrane-coated milk-fat globules and spaghetti-and-meatballs array of proteins and minerals. Make no mistake, the typical four-dollar gallon of milk is a highly processed food.

One could write a book—and many have—about the political maneuvers that led to the current reality that most US states require that milk be pasteurized. One could write another book about the biological consequences of drinking processed milk versus raw. Suffice it to say, raw milk is better for you. It builds stronger bones, is easier to digest (even for many previously dairy intolerant people), and contains more nutrition that is more bioavailable.

Still, you can't just drink raw milk from anywhere. You really *really* need to do your homework. Tainted milk can contain pathogens such as brucella, listeria, and invasive E. coli. Raw milk must come from a trusted source, from a dairy committed to cleanliness, protocol, and animal welfare.

The best time of year to introduce yourself to raw milk varies depending on your local climate. You want the animals to be eating fresh, growing grass because that's their natural food and they will be healthier. Best of all, the milk will taste delicious and the cream to die for. (I add extra cream to my milk and it's as good as ice cream.)

If the idea of raw milk scares you, think of it as *fresh* milk, as in back-on-the-farm with rolling green hills and the scent of grandma's apple pie wafting across the porch. If that doesn't sell it, then at least introduce yourself to the wonders of raw milk cheese, which tend to be far more complex tasting than those made with pasteurized milk, and can be found just about anywhere—even your local warehouse store. Raw cheeses are required by law to be aged long enough to kill bacteria.

(27)
Buy yoghurt.

If there's no suitable fresh milk in your area, the next best thing is organic, whole milk yogurt, preferably from pasture-raised cows. Buy plain, not flavored, which is loaded with too much sugar. The beneficial bacteria that culture milk into yoghurt remediate much of the damage done by pasteurization and homogenization. What's more, because microbes digest most of the lactose sugar, many lactose intolerant people can enjoy yoghurt.

(28)

Buy naturally fermented pickles, sauerkraut, kombucha, and kimchee.

Fermented foods are abundant in traditional cuisines. Real pickles are fermented. So is traditionally made sauerkraut and kimchee. Kombucha is a fermented tea with origins in ancient Russia. There are many more fermented foods out there, but they are harder to find. These four are available in most health food stores. Like yoghurt, their raw ingredients are transformed by microbial activity from something simple to something more complex.

Fermented foods may be a new concept to some people, but they are worth knowing about. Medical research has just begun to understand how battalions of these probiotic microbes living in our tummies are able to protect us from infection by rogue, pathogenic organisms. The more good guys we've got in our intestinal tract, the more military muscle protects us against invasion when bad guys show up, and the better we resist infection. It's that simple.

In *Deep Nutrition*, I describe many digestive benefits associated with eating live-culture fermented foods. Probiotic organisms help to keep things moving through our middles in a timely manner by releasing hormones that help to coordinate a smooth peristaltic action. This may be why some people suffering from chronic bowel pain and inflammation (a.k.a. leaky gut, or "candida") feel better when they eat probiotic foods.

While around the world, people eat fermented foods on a regular basis, in America, their complex flavors and powerful health benefits are only just beginning to be appreciated.

(29)

Don't think tofu is a health food.

Times were, soy was always fermented, a necessary process to both break down otherwise harmful soy-estrogens and thyroid-gland irritants and to significantly boost nutrient content.

Few would consider white flour a particularly healthy form of wheat. Likewise, bland, store-bought tofu is not a particularly healthy form of soy. It is a refined form of a raw ingredient that, like white flour, represents mostly empty calories. It does not deserve to be considered a health food.

If you find the real, traditionally fermented stuff, I recommend you get it—it's loaded with vitamin K and magnesium, and adds pungent complexity to stir fries. Otherwise, if you really enjoy the taste, buy the usual stuff. Just don't call it a health food.

(30)
Buy sprouted-grain breads.

Breads come in a variety of health grades. White bread is least healthy, containing mostly empty calories. Brown bread is often no better, often made from white flour and colored and labeled as wheat. Whole grain is a step up from that. If you want to find where the upper crust of the healthy bread world hang out, head to a health food store, where you can find sprouted-grain bread, a hearty-textured treat.

Sprouted-grain breads are better than whole grain for two main reasons. First, some of the starch (empty calories) has been enzymatically converted into better things, like amino acids, vitamins, and fiber. This conversion reduces the calorie content by 30 to 40 percent. Second, grains lock up their minerals in storage to be released during germination. Sprouting makes these minerals available to you. The presence of all these nutrients makes sprouted grain breads very susceptible to molding, and that's why you find them for sale in the freezer section. If you can't find sprouted grain, or you just don't like it, sourdough is a good alternative.

A word on gluten. Unless labeled "gluten-free," most bread will probably contain gluten. If you have antibodies to gluten, read the ingredients. I understand that a growing number of parents have concerns that gluten may be causing autism. Without dismissing those concerns, I can tell you that at present I find no compelling evidence to support this hypothesis within the articles published to date (including those on caseomorphins and related compounds).

(31)
Buy truly free-range animal products.

There are all kinds of benefits to allowing cows, pigs, and chickens to live in an open, uncrowded, and healthy environment. Not only does having access to the natural forage their bodies and digestive systems were designed for significantly reduce the stress on the animals, the practice guarantees that what winds up on your plate will be far healthier for you. With the growing consumer interest in animal welfare, many stores now stock products labeled "free-range."

Here's the rub: Just as with the term "organic," many dishonest food producers and their attorneys have invented all sorts of novel ways to get around adhering to the spirit and intent of these terms. Most cattle ranchers "finish" their "grass-fed" cattle on corn for 90 days or longer in an effort, they say, to improve marbling. But these practices open the door to abuse, allowing the cattle only a scant few weeks or months on pasture. "Free-range" chickens and turkey may be given access to a tiny, shared plot of grass so that their ability to eat grubs and insects and engage in normal behaviors is negligible. Once you experience the real thing, you'll be able to see and taste the difference.

If you don't already seek out—and yes, pay more—for quality products, then please familiarize yourself with the brutal and unnatural conditions under which feedlot animals are typically raised.

(32)

Meats with bone and skin are better than boneless and skinless.

If you are trying to cook healthier meals for your children, you have to compete with McNugetts, Big Macs, and Taco Bell. They've got an arsenal of artificial flavoring agents on their side. Bland, desiccated chicken breast sprinkled with Mrs. Dash isn't likely to help you win this contest.

To lure them back, you need flavor. But flavors may never develop when you're buying boneless, skinless, low-fat cuts. To get savory-tasting meats, you can buy cuts with bone still in and fat (and for poultry, skin) still on. Bones, skin, and fat not only provide valuable nutrients, they protect the meat while cooking and allow for a richer, juicier, more satisfying dish.

(33)
Know the provenance of your food.

Which wine is better: The one that says California on the label or the one that says Napa Valley? Napa is a specially recognized appellation known worldwide for producing superior reds and whites. Napa wine producers are proud to identify the very vineyard from which they came. Source is part of their brand.

Likewise, cheese that comes from "sheep grazing the hillsides surrounding Rome," as my favorite cheese for grating does, is going to be much better than your average store-brand Parmesan. The more specific the maker can be, the more likely the product is to be of excellent quality.

(34)
Buy local and seasonal.

These buzzwords are not just for people counting their carbon footprints. Buying local helps to ensure freshness, and buying seasonal helps to promote a more varied diet. One of the easiest ways to do both is to shop at your local farmers' markets, the schedules for which are usually posted online by your local farm associations and cooperatives—organizations I like to support.

In his book *Think Like a Chef*, culinary superstar Tom Coliccio tells his readers that the first step to cooking like a pro is to think in terms of seasonality, and then build your menu around those foods that are at their peak.

(35)
Buy quality sauces and salsa.

Your grandmother would never put corn syrup in spaghetti sauce or salsa. Food giants do this as a matter of course. Make your own, or choose the brands with the least amount of sugar. (Compare grams of sugar per serving size.) And if they contain oil, make sure it's a good one (see Rule 3).

(36)
Buy quality condiments.

Off-the-shelf mayonnaise is mostly vegetable oil; ketchup and relish, mostly sugar. Avoid these. Put mustard on your sandwiches instead of mayo, and use tomatoes or real pickles instead of the other two. There are some bad mustards out there, and lesser mustards list sugar and/or some kind of preservative as an ingredient.

(37)

Don't buy foods that make health claims.

If a product suggests it's healthy, it's probably not. Some of the healthiest foods in the store are in the produce section, where few health claims are found simply because the products lack packaging to print on. As Michael Pollan says, don't take the silence of the yams as a sign they have nothing valuable to say about your health.

Along those lines, don't choose foods just because the package tells you it contains fiber, antioxidants, phytonutrients—or whatever the buzzword du jour happens to be. It's the same processed junk it was before, only now it contains a few grams of cellulose (in the case of fiber), or dehydrated fruit and/or vegetable matter (in the case of antioxidants and phytonutrients).

Don't buy products displaying these terms:

- Low-fat
- Low-salt
- High-fiber
- Antioxidants
- Phytonutrients

(38)
Buy smart desserts.

If you taste a bite of dessert and think, "Gosh, that's sweet," then it's not a dessert; it's a formed pile of sugar. Dessert doesn't have to be cloying. Overtly sweet foods are called sickly sweet for a reason—they make you sick. With any dessert, most of the calories should come from healthy fats, and fewer than fifty percent of the calories per serving should come from sugars or other carbohydrates.

Choose these desserts:

- Chocolate: Made with cocoa butter, butter, cream, or palm oil, not vegetable oil or anything hydrogenated
- Ice cream: Made with cream, not milk protein solids
- Cookies: Made with butter, not vegetable oils, and with a very short ingredients list
- Cakes and pies: Cheesecake, crème brûleé, custards, and fruit pies are the best choices. (When making your own fruit pies, don't add sugar to the fruit filling)

(39)
Get great food free: Grow your own!

If you've never grown anything, you'll be amazed how herbs thrive on a windowsill. Especially cooperative are basil, mint, rosemary, bay leaf tree, savory oregano, dill, and chives. These potent sources of fresh antioxidants jazz up any meal.

Part Two: How Should I Cook? (According to tradition)

Many people assume eating healthy means giving up favorite foods like pizza, bacon, fries, coffee, and beer. These foods all belong to an authentic culinary tradition and, when prepared according to traditional methods, are part of a healthy diet. On the other hand, the nutritional value of such supposedly healthy favorites as fish and salads can be diminished by improper cooking techniques and the use of non-traditional ingredients or combinations.

In this section, you will learn to transform the healthy ingredients you bought in Part One into satisfying meals, sometimes in minutes. Your diet will be lower in carbohydrates than the average American's, and far richer in healthful fats and fresh vegetables. Any meat, poultry, or fish you eat will be more nourishing, and you will start enjoying superfoods that you've probably rarely, if ever, had an opportunity to try.

Some of these rules will introduce you to cooking techniques with which your grandmother (or great-grandmother, depending on your age) created what may be the most memorable meals of your childhood. Professional chefs use these same skills to impress the fussiest clientele. Don't worry, though. Just because I've said the words "professional chef" doesn't mean these meals are complicated. All you have to do is follow an orderly sequence of steps in a timely fashion and you'll get where you're going.

(40)
Cook according to tradition.

We all owe our existence to the success of our predecessors' ability to satisfy the twin needs of *staying* alive (by nourishing our bodies) and *feeling* alive (by experiencing pleasure). Happily, the quest for nutrition perfectly complements the quest for flavor, and traditional cooking accomplishes both.

All authentic cuisines use remarkably similar techniques to make full use of the edible local flora and fauna. In *Deep Nutrition* I explain that, as different as Szechuan may seem from Sicilian, *all* authentic world cuisines share the same four categories of food sources and preparative techniques:

Four Pillars of World Cuisine

- Fresh food
- Sprouted and fermented
- Meat cooked on the bone
- Organ meats

These four categories embody ingredients and preparative techniques that are common to cuisines across the globe. Born of pragmatism and ingenuity, they are now built into our DNA. Fresh foods follow seasons. Sprouting and fermenting work with nature, employing the processes of germination and microbial colonization to enhance the nutritional value of the raw material. Cooking can destroy nutrients, but cooking meat on the bone gently and with minimal drying creates the most sinfully savory meals while at the same time protecting the nutrients and providing our bodies with much needed collagen (especially when you save the bones to make bone broth). And organ meats are some of nature's richest vitamin and mineral sources.

Traditional cooking makes best use of your food dollar by honoring the ingredients (paying attention to seasonality, maximizing the "parts" of an animal that can be eaten). Traditional recipes can create sensational meals by simply combining fats with salts or sour with sweet according to time-tested rules. Traditional meals are the vehicles through which our ancestors simultaneously carried enough nutrients into their bodies to survive in a pre-health insurance, pre-government safety-net world while delivering all the joy of flavorful experiences that served as a centerpiece of social life. We can do the same.

(41)

Read one really good cookbook from cover to cover.

With so many recipes available on the web, cookbooks might seem a space-taking redundancy. Many are. But a few stand head and shoulders above the rest:

Five of Luke's favorite cookbooks:

- *The Professional Chef*, Culinary Institute of America
- *Le Cordon Bleu at Home*, Le Cordon Bleu
- *Cooking*, James Peterson
- *The Joy of Cooking*, Irma Rombauer (Buy editions published prior to 1960)
- *Mastering the Art of French Cooking Volume I and II* Julia Child (Buy first edition, recently reprinted. New versions substitute healthy fats with vegetable oil)

These books don't just list recipes. They educate you, providing a crash course in the basics of serious home cooking, everything from how to dress a chicken to how to cut an onion in the least amount of time to how to sharpen a knife. They cover essential traditional cooking techniques from braising and stewing meats and vegetables (matching technique to ingredient) to soup and stock making. All help you master the art of enhancing flavor and maximizing nutrition.

(42)

Involve your kids.

You're not going to want to cook while your kids are screaming, "Where's dinner?!?" My patients tell me this is a big reason they turn to instant meals and fast foods. Once this pattern is established, and you've allowed your children to set the dietary regimen, it can be tough to take the reins again.

What do you do now? Apply a little child psychology.

When I was eight, I couldn't wait for Thanksgiving dinner. Time dragged slowly and I hung around until I drove my mother crazy enough to give me something to do: Slice bread for stuffing. Reluctantly, at first, I piled eight slices and methodically cut them into strips, then little cubes. The chore grew mesmerizing and when the bowl was filled I asked, "What's next?" Before I knew it, I'd made the stuffing all by myself and dinner was now an hour closer. Of course, in the meantime I thought of a few things to do outside.

Rachael Ray grew up watching her mother cook, and started helping in the kitchen as soon as she was tall enough to reach the counter while standing on a chair. Nationally famous talk therapist Dr. Joy Brown often reminds her radio listeners that a child's hierarchy of needs is pretty simple: They want attention. Positive attention is best, but if that's not available, they'll act up to get the bad kind. The worst is to be ignored. Let your kids know that the way to earn your attention is to be helpful in the kitchen, as your "official" sous-chef de cuisine. Give them credit: *Sally made the stuffing*. The passion for cooking begins in childhood. To set them on a track for excellent health, plant the seed early before bad habits take hold.

I'll never forget a study I read in college about the innate ability we have as children to meet our nutritional needs and how that can get lost over time. When allowed to choose among vegetables, fruits, meats, nuts, and dairy, kids naturally gravitate towards a balance that ends up being relatively low in sugar and starch and very healthy. But adults, whose taste buds have often been retrained to crave chips, fries, cookies, and soda, initially eat very oddly. Over time, however, people's taste buds seem to remember themselves and the adults in the study started eating better. (This study was done decades ago, when fewer kids were exposed to the taste-bud altering junk they get today.)

By the way, children traditionally grew up learning all kinds of food-related skills from their parents, helping out with whatever tasks they had developed enough coordination to safely accomplish. These learning experiences strengthen the parent-child bond—and just may inspire a successful career as a culinary artist. Do, please, make sure you review safety tips with your kids whenever you invite them into the kitchen.

Kids or no, if you follow these rules, you will be spending more time cooking. If you have no kids to keep you company, involve your spouse/friends/neighbors or just listen to T.V. or radio. Luke and I spend a lot of time together in the kitchen. He's the head chef in our house, and I still enjoy slicing things into neat little piles.

(43)
Use the right fats and oils for the right jobs.

Including some healthy fat in your meals improves flavor and nutrient bioavailability. With naturally fatty foods such as nuts, cheese, and eggs, you don't need to add extra. But when eating starchy foods or vegetables, adding fat to the meal greatly enhances the nutritional value, protecting heat-sensitive vitamins and antioxidants during cooking, slowing the absorption of sugar into the bloodstream, and optimizing the appropriation of fat-soluble vitamins and nutrients throughout your body.

Here are the two things to consider when choosing which fats and oils to cook with: Fatty acid type, and protein content. Fatty acid type (polyunsaturated, monounsaturated, or saturated) determines how the oil resists oxidation. Protein content determines the smoke point.

Polyunsaturated fatty acids oxidize readily. Once oxidized they become toxic (in much the same way that trans fats are toxic), so oils high in polyunsaturated fat are bad choices for cooking, but fine for salad dressing and dips.

Monounsaturated and saturated fatty acids can handle heat without oxidizing, so fats and oils high in these fatty acids are better choices for frying and baking. Olive and peanut oils, for instance, have a smoke point around 350 degrees Fahrenheit. Refine them, and you remove much of the protein, raising the smoke point by roughly 100 degrees (depending on the grade of refining). Added to all this is the fact that the lower grades of oils have more of the easily oxidized polyunsaturated fatty acids than their first-press counterparts. Unless you have a chemistry degree, it can get pretty confusing. To make it simple, copy the list below and keep it in your kitchen.

You may be surprised to find lard and bacon grease on my list of approved cooking fats. Not so long ago, I had a hard time convincing patients that butter was healthier than margarine—although most could attest to the fact that their grandparents and great-grandparents seemed to thrive on a diet with plenty of butter. For those of you who have known all along that butter and other natural foods win out over food scientists' latest pet creations, I'm happy to say that leading lipid scientists are now backing you up, bringing us back to basics, to real, natural fats and oils and away from vegetable oils, which should be categorically avoided.

Fats and oils for cooking

- Olive
- Butter
- Peanut (especially good when used with small amounts of antioxidant-rich sesame oil)
- Bacon fat
- Coconut
- Palm oil
- Macadamia nut
- Avocado
- Hazelnut
- Lard
- Duck and goose fat

Oils for dressings and dips

- All of the above cooking oils
- Walnut
- Flax
- Sesame
- Wheat germ

(44)
Use fat and salt on veggies.

Vegetables are super-foods that need a little help to bring out their best. Salt or fat, or both together, are just what the doctor ordered.

When eaten without salt or fat, vegetables can taste unappetizingly bitter or bland. That's because most of a plant's flavorful compounds are locked behind microscopic-but-strong cellulose cell walls that our teeth can't bust through. What's more, because flavor ligands are mostly fat-soluble and our saliva contains almost no fat, we can't experience the full flavors of what few juices chewing manages to extract. Cooking and juicing bust through the cellulose barriers, while salt and fat work together to coax the phytonutrients and flavor ligands into direct physical contact with our taste buds. This is no accident of biology. The same salt and fat needed for optimal flavor also facilitate nutrient absorption into the bloodstream. So forcing down bland, fat-free, salt-free greens day after day is as unpleasant as it is unnecessary.

Dip carrot and celery sticks in yoghurt-dill dressing. Scoop roasted red pepper and artichoke tapenade into the cap of a mushroom (or spread over sourdough in place of butter). Butter, sauces, dressings, dips, and spreads are your ticket to getting those three to five servings of veggies each day—and liking it.

Fermented vegetables offer an interesting variation on this rule, as the probiotic organisms, added salt, and lactic acids create additional flavors and aid digestion and nutrient absorption.

(45)
Make a BIG, colorful salad, and dress it right.

Aim for eating salads three or four days a week. The bigger and more colorful, the better. Some of my patients think they're eating salad when it's just five or six leaves of iceberg lettuce and a sliver of tomato. That's not a salad; that's a garnish.

Iceberg and Romaine lettuce aren't as flavorful or nutritious as darker or more bitter leafy greens like arrugula, endive, curly endive, butter lettuce, dandelion greens, red mustard, mizuna, radiccio, chicory, and red rocket (many of these can be found in "mixed baby greens"). Don't stop there. Experiment using beet greens, Swiss chard, collard greens, sliced cabbage, green pepper, celery, carrots, and sprouts. Garnish at will, with various combinations of your favorite things. Mine are pine nuts, cashews or walnuts, capers, raisins, and sprouted or raw sesame seeds.

We eat salads with all different combinations of whatever we have on hand. Each bite combines beautiful colors with pungent, intense, savory and sometimes sweet taste sensations. After pouring on the dressing, add a tablespoon of brine from either the pickle or sauerkraut jar. Probiotics in the brine seed your GI tract with an infusion of microbes that will help digest all this roughage.

If you top your salad with low-fat or no-fat dressing, you may end up flushing most of the fat-soluble vitamins and phytonutrients down the drain. The natural fatty acids present in cream, yoghurt, and olive oil, for example, facilitate absorption.

(46)
Steam and stir-fry vegetables.

The simplest way to prepare vegetables is to assemble them into a large salad. Beyond that, you want to perfect these two super easy techniques. With both, the veggies are done when still just a little bit crunchy.

Frozen vegetables should be rinsed with warm water and allowed to thaw for optimal cooking. Many have already been partially or fully cooked and all you need to do is reheat. I reheat frozen peas, for instance, with butter in a saucepan and then add salt.

Get your greens fast:

- Steam and drizzle with garlic butter and salt. Works well for broccoli, string beans, collard greens, chard, carrots, kale, and cauliflower.

- Stir-fry in peanut oil and, for the last few seconds, a mix of fish sauce, oyster sauce, and that ubiquitous red sauce you see in oriental restaurants known as "Rooster" sauce. Works well with bok choy, string beans, snow peas and pod peas.

- Steam, chill, and drizzle with Italian dressing. Works well with asparagus, carrots, and string beans.

- Sauté in butter. Works well with combinations of two or more of the following: zucchini, tomato, onion, mushrooms, red peppers, and corn. (Zucchini, onion, red pepper, and mushroom taste best if you give them fifteen minutes or more at low heat on the stovetop.)

(47)
Cook meat gently.

Forget the idea of cooking fat out of your meat. Overcooking meat makes it bad for you. Here's why:

Overcooking fuses nutrients and creates toxic Frankenstein molecules. One of the most well studied is heterocyclic amines, highly carcinogenic compounds produced by heating protein in the presence of iron. Water and saturated fat delay these harmful reactions, and this is one reason it's a bad idea to try and cook the fat out. Another is the fact that it just doesn't work. Most of the liquid you see dripping from the meat is water and blood; the burnt fatty acids fuse right into the desiccated flesh and you eat them. If the meat you buy comes from a feedlot, however, depending on the cut you may be better off erring on the side of overcooking (especially with burgers) than risking serious E. coli. As a side note, restaurants tend to serve the least-fresh cuts of meat to people who order well done.

I advise my patients to buy quality meat and cook it gently. If the cut is tough, slow-cooking techniques like stewing and braising will make it savory and delicious. Because the water prevents overheating, these traditional methods are one way to optimize the nutritional value of many of the less costly but extremely healthy cuts. When grilling fillets and other steaks, stop at rare or medium rare.

How to prepare grass-fed steak:

- Marinate your steak for between 30 minutes and a day or so. We marinate in a mix of Worcestershire sauce, olive

65

oil, and fresh ground pepper. (I don't worry about the little bit of sugar and "natural flavorings" in the Worcestershire.)

- Never cook steak straight out of the fridge. By the time the center is heated, the rest is overdone. Let the steak continue to marinate on the counter for about twenty minutes before putting it on the heat.
- Go from high heat to low, never low to high. Sear your steak on both sides to seal in the juices for a minute or so at high heat, then turn the heat way down and allow it to cook slowly.
- Let it rest five minutes before slicing. This allows carryover cooking and permits the juices to be reabsorbed back into the meat.

Even gently cooked meat contains some oxidized fat and amino acid reaction products, and eating meat can be hard on your kidneys because of this. So what's a health-conscious chef to do? Bone stock helps your body use protein to build bones and joints more effectively and seems to protect us from some of the harmful compounds that inevitably develop in even gently cooked meat. The more meat you eat, the more you need stock. So top that gently cooked steak with delicious demi-glace (French for gravy) made by reducing homemade bone broths to about one-eighth their original volume. Adding mushrooms, onions, butter, salt, or whatever you like best, adds five-star flavor to your meat dishes (see next Rule).

(48)
Make bone broth.

According to Julia Child, without sauces "your food is bland, even institutional, while with them you are really cooking." And how do we make sauces? From bone broth. Broth is the cornerstone of cuisines across the globe.

I consider bone broth a missing food group. Made from bones with a cartilage coating at the ends, broth infuses your blood with molecules of collagen and glycosaminoglycan that affect your body in amazing ways. Researchers now use collagen hydrolysate (*hydrolysis* means breaking a protein apart using water molecules) to grow brand new organs from stem cells (stem cells are baby cells that can grow up to be any type of cell). In your body, these molecules travel to worn-out tissues where they make stem cells more plentiful, effectively reversing time in your tissues. This gives bone broths an ability to rejuvenate all your worn-out bones, joints, connective tissues, and the structural supports for skin. Most of these tissues have a low blood supply and would otherwise be unable to heal. Supplements containing glucosamine and chondroitin provide two members of this family of miraculous molecules, but bone stock contains the whole family and works much better.

It doesn't matter what *kind* of animal; all bones can be used to make broth: chicken, pig, cow, fish, etc. What matters is *how the animal was raised*. Animals allowed to move about and enjoy their natural diet build healthier bones and joints. Their bones and joints will become your bones and joints, so you need them to be as healthy as possible.

Bone broth (or *stock*) is made by slowly simmering lightly roasted bones (or bones cooked as part of a meal, as with Thanksgiving turkey, or chicken drumsticks) together with vegetables and some kind of acid to help leach out the minerals (vinegar, wine, tomatoes). The boiling time depends on the diameter of the bones. Cow bones take longer than pig bones, which take longer than chicken, which take longer than fish. Broth wiggles like Jell-O when cool. And the more collagen and glycosaminoglycan you've extracted, the stiffer it gets when chilled. Luke follows a recipe from *The New Professional Chef*, but there are scores of great recipes and instructional videos online. (Most commercially available broths are made just with meat, not bones, and therefore won't provide the same benefits.)

When you don't have time to make stock, do what world-class chef Jacques Pepin does and save the drippings left over from a beef roast or roast chicken. Use water or wine to remove every last bit of juice from the pan, then chill, remove the fat and store in the freezer. Chefs never waste this flavorful, gelatinous liquid gold, and neither do we.

I tell my patients with growing children or any joint or musculoskeletal issue to always keep some kind of bone stock in the freezer and find an excuse to eat some at least two or three times a week, and more often if you eat meat every day.

How we use bone broth:

- As a base for chile, stews, and all soups, instead of water
- In rice, instead of water
- Added to caramelized onions and/or sautéed mushrooms and reduced down to a thick sauce for over our steaks
- In and on mashed potatoes

(49)
Explore different cuisines.

Tired of the same old breaded chicken breast? Try an Indian version: tandoori chicken. Sick of simple noodle soup? Make it Thai style: thom-ka-guy (flavored with coconut and lemon grass). Fed up with eggs and sausage? Head for the border: Buy soft, white corn tortillas (made without vegetable oil), salsa (or make your own in five minutes), organic cheddar cheese, and sour cream, and assemble your own open-face burrito. The theme here is to start with recipes you're comfortable with and perishables you already buy, and expand your repertoire with new herbs and spices from different regions of the world.

Find a dish you really love at any authentic "ethnic" restaurant you can find, and then, with the guidance of a recipe, try to replicate those flavors at home.

(50)
Cook a variety of meats.

One thing all truly traditional diets have in common is that they are not limited to an exclusive list of "premium" cuts. To the contrary, they use everything, from gizzards and giblets to hooves and feet. These "lesser" cuts are typically richer in collagen or other nutrients and, when properly prepared, far more flavorful than the more expensive meats.

Eating snout-to-tail is not only good for you, it's good for the health of your local food chain. If consumers insist on using only premium cuts, they leave the farmer with a surplus of flanks and roasts and rounds and organ meats and bones. One rancher I spoke with told me he couldn't supply a local meat shop because the retailer would only buy the premium cuts. These smaller farms often fail because they can't compete against the mega-industries who sell their own unwanted cuts in bulk lots to hamburger meat and pet food manufacturing companies.

Cuts and parts you can buy cheap:

Beginner
- Brisket
- Belly
- Shoulder
- Round
- Roast
- Skirt, flat iron, and hanger steak

Advanced
- Cheek
- Marrow bones
- Heart
- Kidney
- Liver
- Tongue

(51)
Explore different cooking techniques.

We Americans are fixated on recipes. We collect cookbooks mainly for their recipes, and patients are always asking me about which recipes I recommend.

I recommend you be less focused on recipes and think more like a chef. Most chefs don't memorize recipes but rather perfect a set of techniques, the general principles and methodologies that can be applied to almost any ingredient. This is the true art of cooking. Tougher meats and root vegetables are transformed by braising, for example, while lean meats like chicken breast benefit from marinating and stir-frying. Thomas Keller, perhaps America's best living culinary artist, slowly caramelizes onions for eight hours to turn them into the masterpiece that is his French onion soup.

Not that you need to spend your Saturday stirring an onion in a pot. I tell you this merely to encourage you to have some fun in the kitchen, to experiment with simple techniques applied to a variety of familiar foods.

Basic Techniques for Preparing Meats and/or Vegetables

- Marinating
- Braising
- Poaching and steaming
- Slow cooking and roasting
- Stir-frying
- Grilling
- Caramelizing
- Stewing

(For sauces and gravies to accompany these dishes, see Rule 48.)

(52)
Learn online.

Medical students learn by the axiom *See one, do one, teach one*. Not because our enthusiasm for procedures makes us reckless, but because visual learning is such an incredibly powerful teaching tool that our learning curve is steep. And now, thanks to YouTube, we can all enjoy a culinary learning curve that is equally steep. Of course, you can watch more than one; there are so many great demonstrations on streaming video now that you can see dozens and dozens of variations if you want to get comfortable before attempting a new technique yourself. You'll find everything from "how to make natural peanut butter," to "how to dress a turkey," to "how to caramelize an onion," to "how to grill a perfect NY Strip."

If you're just looking for a recipe and not a technique, a great way to find wonderful recipes online is by typing a traditional cooking implement or technique and a culinary ethnicity into the search window, along with key ingredients. For instance, try: Whole chicken, German recipe, baked. Or: Lamb shanks, English recipe, Dutch oven. Or: Bone stock, brown (for beef broth), French recipe. The other benefit of online recipe hunting comes from the ratings and comments, which can give you a much better idea of what to expect.

(53)
Avoid crummy recipes.

A good guide to an unhealthy recipe or a non-traditionally trained chef is the presence of an industrial product in the list. Rather than make substitutions, better to avoid the recipe entirely.

Don't cook with:

- Non-stick cooking spray
- Margarine or shortening
- Anything with the words "non-fat"
- Any of the vegetable oils
- Canned soups
- Splenda or other artificial sweeteners
- Salt substitutes
- Corn chips
- Corn flakes, raisin bran, or other cereals
- Bacon bits
- Ketchup (this is a major sugar source, only use as a condiment, not a main ingredient)
- Hot dogs (sausage is so much better)
- Mixes (like muffin mix, biscuit mix, etc.)
- A microwave oven

(54)
Cook eggs gently.

Eggs are a very convenient, low-cost superfood. The yolks are nuggets of brain-building phospoholipids, biotin, and choline. Eggs from hens allowed to walk freely and forage for insects and other natural foods are even richer treasures, providing omega-3, and vitamins A and D. But all of these delicate molecules can be destroyed by cooking (and during encapsulation into brain-health supplements). All yolks will be better for you if you leave them runny when possible, and be sure not to scorch when scrambling. Never cook yolks to that dry, crumbly state that makes them pasty and hard to swallow.

The white contains anti-nutrients designed to help protect the developing embryo and so, rather unlike the yolk and most other protein-rich foods, egg whites are more nutritious when cooked because cooking (or whipping) the whites just enough to turn from clear to white deactivates the anti-nutrients.

How many eggs can you eat? Dr. Larry Kaskel, founder of the Heart Attack Prevention Center at Lake Forest, Illinois, explains that, in spite of the common myth that eggs are unhealthy, studies show that people who eat as many as twelve eggs per week are in *better* health than people who don't eat any.

Healthiest ways to cook an egg:

- Poached
- Soft-boiled (hard-boiled are fine for on-the-go meals)
- Sunny and runny

(55)
Make sauerkraut.

If you are ready to join the growing ranks of kitchen tinkerers who have mastered the art of fermenting their own foods, start with sauerkraut, one of the easiest fermented foods to make.

Using a food processor or a good knife, shred a head of cabbage. Then, in a big bowl, mix cabbage with a heaping teaspoon of salt and a tablespoon of the liquid from your favorite fermented pickles (my brand is Bubbies). Pack into a metal or glass container and press down until the water drawn out by the salt covers the cabbage. Place a clean, weighted plate over the top and you're done. Cover with cheesecloth to keep the insects out.

Now, all you need to do is wait. In Hawaii, it took a week. In colder climates, it can take a month or longer. With a spoon or clean paper towel, periodically remove any mold that grows on the surface. You know it's done when it's sour tasting and the cabbagey crunch is pretty much gone. When you have extra cucumbers, you can make pickles by a similar method.

If you find you have a knack with this, or you find yourself swimming in extra vegetables from your garden, expand your repertoire. Just about everything can be fermented, and if you have a bumper crop, this is a far more nourishing preservation method than canning. (There are all sorts of fermentation recipes and videos available for free on the web.)

Before the invention of electricity and refrigeration, knowledge of fermentation represented a critical skill-set, enabling families to put food by for use during winter or times of hardship. Unlike cooking with fire, some kind of fermentation happens all by itself in any food left to sit, and some experts suggest it may be an even older, and therefore more physiologically important, method of food preparation.

Keep in mind that most of those probiotic microbes will be killed if you cook them, so you should eat some live-culture foods raw as side dishes or condiments. (Hard cheeses such as cheddar and Parmesan have been aged to the point that they contain no live cultures.) Still, be sure to experiment, using them in soups (sauerkraut soup) and baked dishes (sauerkraut and cream cheese instead of ricotta in lasagna), because they really do add incredible complexity and exquisite taste sensations.

(56)
Eat raw fish.

Fish are best for us when wild-caught and uncooked. Traditional cuisines typically include raw and pickled or fermented fish as regular staples. Heat destroys nutrients, most notably antioxidants and certain fats and proteins, and animal flesh is rich in all three. The beneficial omega-3 fats are particularly susceptible to the damaging effects of heat and anything above the temperatures of a gentle poaching can begin to destroy them.

Fish suitable to be eaten raw come from salt water, not fresh, have been carefully inspected for parasites by the fish monger, and are typically frozen at temperatures adequate to destroy parasites.

Most of the world's long-chain omega-3 fatty acids originate in the diatomaceous life upon which all other sea creatures feed. These long-chain omega-3 fatty acids are required for normal brain development, and there is no plant that provides them. As I write this, the Gulf is being poisoned with thousands of barrels of oil each day, destroying sea life faster than at any period in recorded history, making it all the more important for us to appreciate and honor the few remaining sources of these crucial nutrients.

Easy, fishy meals:

- Herring in wine or cream sauce (Grocery deli section)
- Poke (Sold in grocery delis across Hawaii)
- Sushi (Available in grocery stores everywhere)
- Mexican-style cheviche

(57)
Avoid protein drinks.

I warn weight lifters, body builders, and everyone who uses protein powders, drinks, and bars that they would be far better off with real food than any supplemental protein products. No matter what health claims you see on the label, all such protein products are concentrated sources of free amino acids, which can bind to collagen in your connective tissues very much like sugar can, so all these products have potentially corrosive effects on your joints and other tissues.

Besides the obvious protein powder products, there are a dazzling number of protein additives, all with the same potentially harmful effects. They go by many names, but all are combinations of one or more of these three terms: protein, extract, and hydrolyzed, with one of these: soy, yeast, casein, or vegetable. Sometimes they call it "natural flavorings."

If you want to drink supplemental protein, make yoghurt smoothies, eggnog with real egg yolk (from safe sources), and soup. Keep in mind, however, that too much of anything, even protein, can be bad. With the popularity of low-carb, low-fat, high-protein diets, I've seen people developing joint and blood pressure problems that I believe stem from connective tissue damage due to excessive lean meat consumption.

(58)
Make your own salad dressing.

People sometimes switch out starchy dishes for salads and are surprised that they don't lose weight. In some cases, cholesterol and triglyceride numbers climb, and liver enzyme counts get worse.

The problem is the dressing.

As I mention in Rule 13, salad dressings (this includes dressings and mayonnaise that say "made with olive oil") may also contain both vegetable oil and sugar, which disrupt your metabolism. Your physician may presume you are genetically predisposed to bad health and insist you take a cholesterol pill.

Here's what I recommend: Make yourself a nice balsamic vinaigrette dressing:

    2/3 cup extra virgin olive oil (the best are green and cloudy)
    1/3 cup balsamic vinegar
    1/2 tsp honey
    2 tsp salt
    1 tsp Dijon or stone ground mustard
    3 cloves garlic
    1 shallot, or 1/4 onion
    1 tsp bacon fat (optional, delightful)
    Italian spices (I use fresh oregano, thyme, and basil)

Put everything except the olive oil in a blender and then slowly drizzle in the olive oil through the little hole in the blender lid while the blender is running.

(59)

Make soup.

If any food embodies a mother's love it has to be soup. The smell of soup simmering, the warmth of a bowl in your hands, the fullness in your belly—everything about soup is wonderful. The secret to extraordinary soup is to start with bone stock, rather than water, for a base.

Soup can take half a day or more to make, but it stores and freezes well and, with practice (and a good slow cooker or crock pot), you can streamline the workflow, make giant batches, and, depending on family size, live on leftovers for the rest of the week.

Soups we make:

- Chicken and dumpling (chicken stock)
- Split pea, ham, and bacon with potatoes (chicken stock)
- Green chile with roasted green chile peppers and ham (chicken stock)
- Thai chicken soup with lemon grass and coconut called *thom ka gai* (chicken stock)
- Beef barley (beef stock)
- Oxtail soup (beef stock)
- French onion (beef stock)
- Chile con carne and sprouted beans (beef stock)
- Vegetable medley (beef or chicken)
- Vietnamese pho (beef or chicken)
- Filipino-style salmon head soup (salmon bones are small enough that no added stock is needed)

(60)
Become a flavor junkie.

I don't know how it happened that people started associating blandness with healthfulness. I particularly remember a kindly patient of mine who clearly hoped I'd be impressed by the fact that she ate plain water crackers for lunch. Always remember: Flavor equals nutrition. I don't want you ever thinking you have to give up good-tasting foods.

As long as we're not talking about MSG or other fake ingredients, the more flavor a food has, the healthier it is. (More flavor indicates a higher nutrient-to-calorie ratio.) This doesn't just apply to different kinds of foods, it also holds true when comparing, say, one cucumber to another—the more "cucumbery" one is healthier.

If you don't enjoy goji, acai, turmeric, or whatever today's superfood may be, don't trouble yourself hunting them down. The old-school superfoods, like garlic, ginger, green pepper, celery, and mustard greens, are just as good. What all these foods share is an intensity of flavor. All that taste comes from a super-concentration of different anthocyanins, polyphenols, flavonoids, alkaloids, anthraquinones, and other phytonutrients.

The taste test also applies to meats, cheeses, and even wine. Meat and cheeses will reflect the animal's diet: Bland silage cannot compare in terms of taste or nutrition to the green, leafy forage healthy cows get. A good red wine contains more bioflavonoids (including resveratrol) than an insipid white. If your diet feels repetitive and boring, you're on the wrong track—if you can't taste much, there's not much there for your cells to use.

(61)

Don't cook. Find ready-to-eat foods made only with natural ingredients.

Not everyone has time to cook every meal themselves. Thankfully, the more conscientious food stores consistently stock healthy ready-to-eat meals.

Look for soups, salads, sauces, frozen entrees, and other prepared foods that use healthy fats (olive or peanut oils, cream or butter) and don't contain vegetable oil, corn syrup, MSG, or artificial ingredients. Some grocery stores making their own on-site are insisting on quality—and often local—ingredients. You might have to ask what kinds of oils are in the deli salads to find out. If they don't know, presume it's canola or another vegetable oil and don't buy—and tell them why.

(62)
Eat liver.

Organ meats are some of the richest sources of nutrients that are otherwise missing from our diets. Of all the organ meats, liver is the most readily available in grocery stores. You can buy chicken, duck, and cow's liver, liver pâtés, and liverwurst. Pâtés and liverwurst on toast with mustard make for easy, super healthy meals.

People often ask: *Isn't liver full of toxins?* The liver will reflect the quality and content of the animal's diet, just like the animal's fat, flesh, other organs, and even bones. I recommend eating cow or chicken livers from animals given access to the outdoors and their natural forage (no sunlight means no vitamin D in their tissues), fed only limited soy or corn feed, and given no unnecessary antibiotics, hormones, or other unnatural chemicals.

<u>Sandy's Miracle Liver Recipe:</u>

I include this one organ meat recipe to show that you can get these slimy tidbits to taste good and it doesn't take a culinary arts degree. This Filipino adobo-style (marinated in soy sauce) dish is my friend Sandy's own creation. Her children love it and so do we!

Ingredients
1 cow's liver, cleaned (about one pound)
or 1 pound of chicken livers
4-6 cloves garlic

1/8 cup soy sauce (naturally brewed, not hydrolyzed)

2-4 Tbsp Olive or peanut oil

Pepper

Prep and cooking time: 20 minutes

Serves 3 to 4

How to Make

Using a sharp chef's knife, dice the garlic and set aside. If using cow's liver, slice into one inch cubes. Pour oil into a large, flat-bottomed frying pan, coating the bottom, turn heat to medium, toss in the garlic and heat until it starts to sizzle. Sauté garlic a few seconds, stirring. Add liver and cook briefly on each side until evenly brown and blood starts oozing out, about two to three minutes. It should smell savory and good by this point.

Working quickly, grind very generous amounts of black pepper over the meat, about 1/4 to 1/2 tsp, then add the soy sauce into the pan, not pouring over the liver (to avoid washing off the pepper) and place a lid over the top. Turn off heat, leave on hot stovetop and let sit for five to ten minutes until the blood turns pale brown. Serve au jus (that's what we do), over rice, or over noodles with a sprinkle of Parmesan cheese. Oddly enough, this liver will also taste good the next day!

(63)

Don't make a meal out of sugar.

There's sugar added to so many products these days, it's especially important to avoid making it the main ingredient in your meals. One of the benefits of cooking from scratch at home is that you can avoid being smothered in the usual avalanche of sugar in products like barbecue and pasta sauce, salsa, and salad dressing.

Other sugar sources you may not have suspected:

- Peanut butter: Get the kind with an oily layer on top. Most national brands are loaded with sugar, which sops up all the oil.
- Jelly and Jam: Choose brands that contain less than 10 grams of sugar per serving. Top-quality spreadable fruits will have even less than that.
- Rice, soy, and almond milks: Most of these are sweetened with evaporated cane juice or other sugars.
- Energy bars: Treat as cookies.
- Coffee confections and energy drinks: Don't mix addictive substances; if you need caffeine, don't sweeten it.

Don't worry about a blood sugar bump from non-starchy foods that aren't particularly sweet, such as carrots and milk. Almost all plant parts contain some sugar, but in my view, if a natural product doesn't taste really sweet, those sugar molecules are not present in concentrations that will cause you any trouble.

(64)
Eat bitter things.

You've probably heard of the health benefits of kale, turmeric, and red wine. What do they all have in common? Bitterness—the astringent sensation that makes you press the back of your tongue to the roof of your mouth when you taste these foods. Modern science is confirming what Ayurvedic practitioners have known for years, that certain flavors translate to specific health benefits, and one of the six celebrated flavors is bitter. So what makes something bitter? As I've said before, intense flavors typically signify intense levels of nutrition. In the case of bitterness, it's antioxidants.

Kale is particularly rich in silforaphane, which has been associated with anticancer properties. Curcumin, in turmeric, associated with fighting infection. Resveratrol, in red wine, associated with heart health. All of these function as antioxidants and none of these foods have the market cornered on healthfulness; *all* bitter-tasting plants have similar benefits. Antioxidants are anti-inflammatory. And since inflammation is at the root of nearly all illness, all bitter-tasting things can help you fight cancer, aging, heart disease, and more.

What sweetness is to baby food, bitterness is to grown up food. Bitterness is the opposite of sweetness in many ways. We are hardwired to appreciate this flavor as we age, and so we naturally seek out those foods richest in the biochemicals that protect us from inflammation and provide a long life. So seek out bitter foods. If you don't eat many raw foods, it is especially important for you to fortify your diet with the antioxidants found in bitter foods.

(65)
Don't cook dinner every night.

Professional chefs work hard—really hard. Those who put in the extra hours to bring us the gift of a healthful and authentic meal should be cherished, encouraged, and given our patronage.

Some of my husband's best dishes were first introduced to us in a restaurant. Then, using a few similar recipes as a guide, Luke would attempt the dish several times, honing in on the "flavor profile" of the inspiring meal. Our favorite restaurants tend to be modest mom-and-pop establishments, the kind with plastic tablecloths and chairs and free of the bling that may be an endeavor to disguise a lack of culinary integrity—and that also drive up costs. (Not that there's anything wrong with a fancy restaurant!)

These questions will identify the best restaurants in town:

1. Do they make their own bone stock?
2. Do they source local ingredients?
3. Do they change their menu based on seasonality?
4. Do they use authentic oils and fats, not vegetable oils and shortenings?
5. Does the chef have a real passion for cooking? (You'll know this when you hear how the hostess/waitress/proprietors answer the other four questions.)

(66)

Buy good knives and keep them sharp.

You can now purchase an excellent set of forged stainless steel knives, complete with a knife block, for under a hundred and fifty dollars. In his book *Knife Skills Illustrated*, Peter Hertzmann suggests that, although it's nice to have a variety of knives in the kitchen, you really only need two for most tasks: a chef's knife and a paring knife. You are better off owning two quality knives than a whole drawer full of junkers. Be especially picky when choosing the chef's knife, the workhorse of the kitchen. There is no other piece of cooking equipment with which you will develop such an intimate and long-lasting relationship.

To keep that relationship on the best of terms, make sure to sharpen and hone your knives. Sharpening, which you only need to do occasionally, puts a sharper edge on the blade but leaves it irregular and wavy. Honing aligns that microfine edge, restoring the knives' ability to cut. So before you start cooking, hone your knife every time.

(67)

Make your kitchen a nice place to work.

Warped pots and pans, a tiny cutting board, dirty workstations, small bowls, and other remnants from your earliest days as an independent adult have no place in a mature kitchen. I already discussed knives, and of course you also need the basic cooking, stirring, and eating utensils, cups, bowls, plates, frying pans, saucepans, and pots.

These essential tools will help make cooking more pleasant:

- Gallon-plus size metal bowls for making salads
- Wire mesh strainers, small, medium, and large
- Colanders, at least one metal (for hot water, etc.)
- A wok
- A large stock pot
- Several generously sized cutting boards, both wood and plastic (dishwasher-safe plastic is best for meats)
- Vegetable peeler
- Coffee grinder (for fresh ground coffee, spices, and wheat flour)
- Large jars for making sauerkraut
- Cheesecloth or linen towels
- A spice ball or tea infuser
- Rolling pin
- Slow cooker, Crockpot, or Dutch oven
- Sharpening stone, 400/1000 grit

Unfortunately, it can be tough to find a good can opener, for instance, without spending about fifteen dollars, but it makes life so much easier. If you're ever replacing your kitchen faucet, get the tallest one you can afford, and a deep stainless steel sink while you're at it. Bottom line: Skimping on kitchen tools and appliances can waste time—and flesh—especially when you're under pressure to get that meal on the table.

(68)
Save the fat.

When Luke or I make bacon, we pour the fat into a little cup and store it in the fridge. It's a delicious substitute for butter in sautéed and fried dishes. When making stock, we save the fat cap that rises to the top once the stock has cooled to use for basting and deep-frying. And we never cut away (free-range) chicken skin.

I shudder when I see TV personalities advising their audience to trim the fat and throw it away. This advice makes sense only in the context of mass-produced feedlot animals whose fat bioconcentrates the toxins used along the entire industrial food chain. As a result, these animals lay down fat full of pro-inflammatory, endocrine-disrupting chemicals that you don't want to eat. So rather than buying substandard meat and trimming the fat away, get meat you can feel good about and make use of that precious, delicious fat.

(69)
Add fresh herbs later than dried.

Dried herbs lose complexity—both in terms of flavor and nutrition—because, during the drying process, the more volatile aromatics evaporate or are oxidized. When cooking with fresh herbs, protect these delicate compounds by subjecting them only to the minimum amount of heat necessary to release their flavorful oils, as little as a minute or two before the dish is finished cooking.

(70)
Sprout whole grains and beans.

In an earlier rule, I mentioned that common, store-bought tofu unfairly benefits from the reputation of real tofu, which is always fermented. Similarly, old world whole grains and beans like quinoa, kamut, and lentils are now riding the coattails of more ancient, traditionally produced versions that were often allowed to germinate before being added to a recipe.

Whole grains and beans, those pellets of starch and protein—as nutritionism has us thinking of them—are actually dormant seeds. They are equipped with a blend of enzymes that, once awakened, miraculously transform a hard kernel into something green and growing and full of amino acids, vitamins, cellulose, and more. By letting nature take its course and germinating seeds before consuming them, your body gets all these nutrients. Whether you like quinoa or wheat berries, garbanzos or pintos, you can shorten cooking times and make healthier meals by sprouting before cooking.

How to Sprout Beans, Wheat Berries, and Other Seeds

- Pour into oversized container (allow room for seeds to triple in size), fill with water, and soak overnight
- Drain into a large strainer, rinse, and place strainer over a bowl so that the bottom has access to air
- Rinse for 30 to 60 seconds once or twice a day (to prevent mold growth) until rootlets are 1/8 to 1/4 inch long

(For recipes and other tips, consider joining one of the many groups of like-minded enthusiasts sprouting up all over the web.)

(71)
Eat pickles with meals.

Previously, I praised pickles for their probiotic powers because, with programmatic consumption, probiotics promote a healthier digestive tract and powerful immune system. However, eating real, fermented pickles (sauerkraut, kimchee, cucumber pickles, pickled beets, etc.) with your meals also has an *immediate* benefit as well: Pickles aid digestion.

Eating pickles with food, just an ounce or two, can be particularly helpful to people with gastritis, acid reflux, and other digestive problems. These GI disorders are characterized by inadequate stomach acid production (the inflamed stomach tries to protect itself by cutting acid production). The acids in pickled foods are not strong enough to exacerbate gastritis but plenty strong enough to activate digestive enzymes in the small intestine. And the salt in fermented foods assists bile acids in dissolving and digesting fats. If you can't find the perfect pickle, any sour, salty food will do.

Part Three: How should I eat?
(Eat Mindfully)

Eating mindfully means knowing, appreciating, and celebrating whatever it is you're putting into your mouth. That means knowing where it came from, who harvested and prepared it, and its place in culinary history. As a happy coincidence, this approach toward the gift of food also helps you get healthy. The rules in this section foster habits that will help you stay healthy for the rest of your life.

To prepare for success, it's important to realize how we've been set up to fail. The reality is that most of us have gotten caught in a dysfunctional relationship with food. My friend Catherine, for example, is a young, fit, beautiful, and confident woman who also happens to be an Olympic medalist with a passion for health and nutrition. But her passion was born of pain: She suffered from bulimia, a serious eating disorder. She once asked me if I thought there was some relationship between our dying culinary traditions and the epidemic of eating disorders in the US. I replied that, in my view, our entire country is suffering from a kind of eating disorder.

It's no wonder. We're afraid of our food. We're worried it's going to make us fatter. We've heard about the weird chemicals it probably contains and how they can cause cancer, or birth defects, or hormone changes. We don't like to think about how it's farmed because we know most of the cows and pigs and chickens we're eating were badly mistreated. We don't even want to imagine where it comes from because most of it is grown in polluted environments or just plain ugly landscapes. And to top it off, our schooling leaves us, as adults, utterly unfamiliar with basic principles of home cooking. Within the context of this dysfunctional relationship with our food, an eating disorder can start to look like an understandable, if not predictable, reaction.

Many health and food writers have investigated the roots of our national eating disorder and, looking to the French as role models, suggest that the secret to health comes not so much from any particular component of a meal (the wine, say, or the resveratrol in the wine) but from a healthy attitude towards the whole of the eating experience. The French don't snack; they luxuriate in communal meals, rarely eating alone or in a hurry. The portions they choose are smaller, and second helpings uncommon. Eating is a celebration, not a chore. All we need do, these writers suggest, is shift our mindset in this direction. I agree completely—but there's still a major piece missing from the puzzle. The essential element of the French Paradox that tends to be overlooked is this: In France, they've got *great* food. It's natural. It's traditional. And it's everywhere—you don't need to belong to a club or search the web to find it.

French farmers, chefs, and artisans (like cheese and winemakers) celebrate traditional methods at every step from field to table, giving the average Frenchman the opportunity to eat great-tasting meals crafted from top-quality ingredients. The tasty selections on the table are more likely to inspire conversations about things like what village the food came from, who grew it, and how the chef worked his magic. The majority of American food producers, in contrast, participate in the industrial food chain where volume and ability to withstand long-distance travel matter more than things like flavor or nutrient content. When a healthy consumer market such as the French enjoy can be replicated in America, our national eating disorder—and its raft of attendant health problems—will begin to resolve on its own.

(72)
Surround yourself with foodies.

These days, if you want to find good food it helps to belong to a club. Lots of people love to eat. Foodies celebrate the art of good eating. This means seeking out fresh and seasonal local ingredients, sharing cooking tips, discovering authentic restaurants and ethnic markets, trying new kinds of foods, and doing all of these with like-minded friends as often as possible. An unavoidable consequence of spending time with people who love real food is improved health.

My favorite foodie groups are those with local chapters.

Great places to find foodies online include:

- Slow Food USA
- Epicurean.com
- localharvest.org
- Your local Organic Farmers Associations (in New England it's NOFA)
- Organic Farming Research Foundation
- Edible Communities

Sometimes these organizations will be off the mark when it comes to vegetable oils and saturated fat. Use these resources not for nutritional advice but rather to learn where to buy the kinds of foods you want and how to master new cooking techniques.

(73)

Focus on the nutrients, not the calories.

For most people the problem is not that they get too many calories (though they often do), it's that they get too few nutrients and their body is telling them to eat more than they should. If you are one of those people who hates the idea of counting calories, weighing portions, or determining what you get to eat next by computer program or a color-coded plastic wheel, then flip the formula on its head. Instead of eating *fewer* calories, eat *more* nutrients.

It goes without saying that if your desire is to eat as many nutrient-dense foods as you can in favor of those foods that lack nutritional power, you'll necessarily be eating fewer *empty* calories—and that's the point. Much of the reason we eat until we're stuffed rather than simply satisfied is because we haven't given our body the nutrients it needs. So listen to your body. Give it what it wants: Nutrient dense foods. Eat them plentifully—but once you feel satisfied, stop eating, and if there's more on your plate, save it for tomorrow.

(74)
Don't snack.

When I was growing up, frequent snacking was seen as something akin to antisocial behavior. Now, snacking appears to be America's most popular hobby. I've even heard well-meaning dietitians advise people to snack for the sake of their health to "prevent their blood sugar from bottoming out." This fad supports the snack-food oriented industrial food chain, which booby-traps offices with tempting plates of junk, makes kids lazy, and undermines everyone's health.

A normal metabolism is more than capable of handling long intervals between feedings. So if you need snacks to regulate your blood sugar, it means your metabolism is already in moderate disarray. Ironically, one of the reasons metabolism gets deranged in the first place is that constant high blood-sugar levels maintained by frequent consumption of high-carb foods disrupts your cells' ability to absorb glucose and respond to insulin signals. If you have weight you'd like to lose and are eating three square meals a day, *there is no such thing* as a healthy snack.

That said, when people with glucose intolerance or diabetes start eating healthier, they may need to eat a small, low-carb meal every two or three hours for a month or so until their cells can utilize insulin better and they can go the four to six hours between meals without feeling sluggish.

(75)
Eat meals.

A meal is everything that a snack is not. While snack foods are typically eaten in isolation—one food all by itself—a meal is composed of a number of different foods. This aids in nutrient absorption from the GI tract and allows a fuller spectrum of nutrients to work synergistically inside the body. People often eat snacks on the go. Eating is supposed to activate your digestive system; rushing around slows it down. So speed-eating sends competing signals, impairing digestion. Finally, people tend to be able to rationalize eating junk during a snack more easily than they can during a meal.

I'd like to address a few myths about the timing of your meals. I've heard it said that going for a walk after eating "burns the energy better." That's not true. After a big meal, the blood supply is being diverted into your digestive system and away from muscle, so while it's fine to go for a gentle stroll after a meal, this is not a time for a calorie-burning workout. We're inclined to feel sleepy after a big meal because blood flow is also diverted away from the brain. So if you've done the dishes already, go off to bed.

A related metabolic myth is that eating just before sleeping forces your body to turn those calories into fat. This myth might be based on the idea that your body is basically dormant during sleep. In reality it's anything but. During sleep your body carries out the majority of its growth and repair, and solidifies the day's learning into long-term memory. I do, however, recommend light exercise or stretching first thing in the morning to kick-start your metabolism (see Doctor's Orders).

(76)
Enjoy pizza, cheeseburgers, and beer.

These foods aren't inherently bad. They've gotten a bad rep because they're mostly manufactured within the industrial food chain using the cheapest ingredients manufactured in the fastest, cheapest, least healthy way. The difference between a fast food pizza and Luke's—with fresh-ground wheat-berry flour in home-made crust, homemade sauce, organic mozzarella, and local sausage—is night and day. If you take the time to make your favorite foods for yourself rather than relying on businesses that just want your money, you can be sure they're made in a way that's good for you.

Making a cheeseburger from grass-fed beef is just as easy as making it from lean, grain-fed ground beef—you should add an egg for fat, and oatmeal to hold it all together. We use sourdough or toasted sprouted grain breads instead of those squishy white buns.

Brewing beer, however, is quite an undertaking. Luke used to brew his own beer, but with so many great local microbrewers, these days it's easier to buy great beer than home brew—leaving more time to make pizza.

Signs of a healthy beer:

- Lots of flavor (gives you antioxidants)
- Unfiltered (yeast remains, a great source of B vitamins)
- Unpasteurized (heat kills B vitamins)

(77)
Plan for chaos.

Many people with weight problems tell me that their biggest pitfall is getting busy and having to grab something in a hurry, and then reaching for junk, usually carbs—food bars, crackers, bread, chips, pretzels, candy, etc. I ask them to plan chaos-compatible breakfasts and lunches. Eat what might be considered a snack, but call it a meal and make it healthy. Figure out what kinds of nutritious things you'd like to snack on, and be sure to always have some around.

Two-minute meal ideas:

- Natural peanut butter on a stick of celery, or a banana, or a halved apple
- Cucumber and tomato slices with balsamic vinegar and dash of salt (or 1 Tbsp pickle juice)
- One ounce of hard cheese with one ounce of raw nuts
- One ounce of soft cheese (i.e., brie) on a small slice of sourdough bread, sliced tomatoes optional
- Smoked oysters on a toasted slice of sprouted grain bread
- Liver pâté on healthy toast, with mustard
- Two ounces of pickled herring and a carrot
- Three to four ounces of pickled (fermented) beets and one or two teaspoons of yoghurt or sour cream
- Hard-boiled egg with sea salt
- Hard-boiled egg with kimchee
- A cup of raw milk with 2 Tbsp raw cream, flavored with 1/4 cup of strong coffee or tea, or blended with a banana

One of the worst American habits is eating junk for breakfast and, thanks to charismatic cartoon characters more widely recognized than American Presidents in some parts of the world, sixty percent of the breakfast-eating population in the US start their day pouring machine-molded starch into their bowl.

Just as easy and infinitely healthier is a yoghurt parfait: 1/2 to 1 cup of plain, full-fat organic yoghurt topped with something to give it crunch and flavor. I use sprouted wheat berries, lots of cream, and coffee (not for everyone, I'm sure). Luke tops his with a shy teaspoon each of jelly and vanilla plus a handful of raw walnuts, cashews, or macadamia nuts—whatever we have around. If you get tired of yoghurt, throw a slice or two of sprouted grain bread in the toaster and then slather with something satisfying, like butter, cream cheese, or peanut butter.

If you've got breakfast under control, master the art of the randomly assembled lunch. Many days I bring a collection of foods to work: an ounce or two of cheese, a peeled carrot or a pickle, a handful of raw nuts, and a kombucha.

These, and the list on the previous page, all work great for me, but the key is to figure out what kinds of things *you* like, good foods that really satisfy you, so you never have to resort to eating stuff you know is nothing but empty calories.

(78)
Don't waste good food.

You might have heard it said that an easy way of portioning better is to leave some food on your plate. This is an outmoded, unsustainable piece of advice born of the post-WW II boom, a time when the Earth and all its bounty were seen as an inexhaustible resource.

The reality is, good food is getting harder to come by. To waste any dishonors all the people who participated in its creation, from the chef and grocer all the way back to the farmer, rancher, or fisherman—and of course the food itself. It sends the message to your children that the stuff you're feeding them isn't that important after all.

Get the doggie bag. Eat the skin. Save the bones for broth. Put a smaller portion on your plate—and drink a whole glass of water *before* you go for that second helping.

(79)

Don't depend on others to feed your children right.

If your kids are like most kids, they are exposed to nothing but highly processed, fattening, and unhealthy food in their school cafeteria. Federal lunch programs limit saturated fat to a tiny ten percent of calories, so most of the calories come from carbohydrates (which will become sugar in the bloodstream), milk is skim (sweetened with more sugar), and they use "cheese food" instead of cheese. The only way your child is going to get the nutrition he or she needs to develop normally is if you give it to them.

I'm not saying it's easy to do, but it can be done. One of my patients on Kauai was a single mom with an hour-and-a-half round-trip commute to and from work. She prioritized her time so she could spend Sundays in the kitchen with her eight-year-old daughter making meals for the coming week from scratch. If you're wondering whether doing this yourself would really be worth the trouble, here are a few medical facts that might help motivate you.

According to the CDC, a child born today stands a roughly one in five chance of becoming obese before graduating high school. Not pudgy. Not a little on the heavy side. Obese. Recent studies indicate that roughly forty percent of obese children suffer from sleep apnea and can expect a significantly lowered IQ as a result of their brain being deprived of oxygen. Check out childhood obesity on the Internet and here is just a sampling of the health consequences you can expect to see: Diabetes, depression, herniated discs, hypertension, heart failure—even stroke.

Fat kids are not fat simply because they lack self-control. The truth is, they can't stop eating because they're starving. Every cell in their bodies is demanding nutrients that never arrive and so they continue to scream out for more. These powerful hunger signals spur a child to seek the intense flavors that in a more natural setting correlate to high nutrient content. On a typical American diet, however, these are provided not in nutrient-dense foods, but in starchy, oily foods like breadsticks, fish sticks, chicken fingers, personal pizza, and hot dogs, all of which are laced with MSG and other taste bud-tricking chemicals. Throw fruit juice, soda, and sports drinks into the mix and you can see what your kids are up against.

They need *you*.

(80)
Keep meal routines exciting.

Most people associate healthy eating with restriction. In reality, the opposite is true. As I write in *Deep Nutrition*, it's limitation that's killing us. Most grocery store items are little more than different combinations of the same three ingredients: vegetable oil, sugar, and starch. What apparent variety we are offered comes only from different shapes, flavoring, and coloring agents. By resolving to leave vegetable oil, sugar, and (most) starches behind, you will have made the first step toward a world of greater diversity.

When Luke and I catch ourselves having the same kind of meals over and over we make a conscious effort to break the doldrums by going to the Internet and finding a totally new recipe to make—but it takes that conscious effort. Whatever diet you're on, if you start to feel bored, don't be drawn back to the three-ingredient, highly restricted diet. Keep moving forward. Become a flavor junkie. Look for new material. Boldly go into new restaurants and attempt new recipes until you've tried every good food there is to try. If you're lucky you'll be doing that for the rest of your life.

(81)

To be sexier, eat sexy foods.

Corn chips aren't sexy. Homegrown sweet corn dripping with real butter is hard to sit near without salivating. Vegetable oil—not sexy. Extra virgin, unrefined olive oil—definitely sexy. "Cheese food" isn't sexy. But a Manchego cheese crafted in the La Mancha region of Spain presents a sense of mystery and excitement.

Here's the quick test to determine what's hot and what's not: Think about a movie that featured food prominently in its story line (*Eat Drink Man Woman*, *Like Water for Chocolate*, *Big Night*). Or imagine a romantic scene in which two lovebirds enjoy a late afternoon picnic at the edge of a shimmering lake. What succulent, enticing, crisp and colorful, fragrant foods might you expect to see?

I know it's unrealistic to say that we can all have sexy foods all the time, but when you can eat sexy, go all the way.

(82)
Eat wild, not farmed.

Expanding human population and development mean that there is less wild anything this year than there was last year, and this includes food—most conspicuously fish, whose populations are falling precipitously. Many salmon species have disappeared completely from the rivers in which they once thrived.

This in turn means that there is no longer enough wild food to go around. It doesn't change the fact, however, that wild foods—fattened on a natural diet or, in the case of plants, healthy soil—are healthier than their cultivated cousins. For example, wild salmon contains far more vitamins, omega-3 fatty acids, and other nutrients than the farmed varieties whose flesh would be grey but for their diet of orange-colored food pellets.

So who gets the wild foods? I hate to say it, but those who can afford it. If you can, be sure to appreciate it too.

(83)
Eat with good intention.

Few of us who eat meat could kill an animal ourselves. As the great spiritual educator Joseph Campbell has said, life is participation in a never-ending cycle of destruction and creation. In our ancestral past, worship included songs, dances, stories, and myths that celebrated mindful participation in the never-ending cycle of life. But today's religions don't address the issue so directly, and many of us who feel bad about eating animals have no elixir for our spiritual indigestion. I think this is why, for many people, once they get an eyeful of ugly images from industrial farms, vegetarianism seems like the right thing to do. The fact remains, however, that if you plan to have children, this is not going to be good for them (for reasons detailed in *Deep Nutrition*).

So now you face a rather unhappy dilemma: Help animals or help your child. Short of heading to Africa and signing up with the Maasai (or other tribal culture with a living mythology), how can we Americans raise the healthiest possible child in a spiritually happy place?

What do I do? I make sure that the domesticated animals I eat have had an easier, more carefree life than they would have had living in the wild. And to do that, I have to get in my car and drive. I go to local butcher shops, farmers markets, and farms, and meet the people who make my dinners possible. When I find a rancher or farmer who talks about caring for animals in ways that make me think he or she actually gives a damn, I know I've found someone who deserves my money.

(84)
Make veggies more filling.

In Part Two, I talk about how healthy fats enhance the flavor and nutrition we get from eating greens. Adding fat to veggies is also a great way to curb the all-American tendency to overeat.

Let's say you lost all sense of self-control. Even if you had unlimited access to food, you would eventually be forced to stop eating for one of two reasons: Either a stuffed belly (mechanical limitation), or nausea (chemical limitation). No matter how much self-control you have, learning to trigger the stop switch will aid in portion control and avoiding unnecessary hunger.

Vegetable bulk (cellulose fiber) physically stretches your gut. This mechanical pressure helps make you feel full. If the veggies are eaten with some salt, the salt draws water into the GI tract, further increasing internal pressure and nudging your belly's mechanical switch closer to its "stop eating now" setting.

Fat, as in the olive oil in Italian dressing, releases *endorphins,* which quash hunger pangs and produce a mellow, satisfied feeling. The cholesterol in animal fats—now we're talking about something like butter or a creamy yoghurt dressing—triggers the release of these chemicals more rapidly than does oil. Cholesterol so effectively binds our brain's chemical satiety chemoreceptor, eating too many eggs (especially if that person is unaccustomed to cholesterol-rich foods), at one sitting, for example, can trigger nausea before a person's belly is halfway full. If you can't put down your fork until compelled by fullness, then combine both methods to trigger a full feeling by both chemical *and* mechanical means.

(85)
Include fat early in the meal.

If you're following the other rules but still find yourself eating more than you'd like, try this simple trick: Swallow a teaspoon of fish or flax oil before a meal.

(86)

Put carbs in their proper place.

It's easy to overeat carbs. Enzymes in your saliva quickly convert starch into sugar, and even a tiny hint of sugar stimulates appetite. In your stomach, digestive juices dissolve the starch so that it takes up relatively little physical space and, unlike most other foods, you can keep eating and eating without feeling full.

Both these qualities make carbs a comfortable way for athletes to pack energy into their body, where the athlete's healthy metabolism will direct it into storage as muscle glycogen. Before running the Philadelphia and Boston marathons, my high school teammates and I scarfed down as much spaghetti as we could.

Carb-loading is great for endurance athletes, not so great for everyone else. Unless your muscles are hungry, those extra calories will be converted to fat and stored under your skin. Not that I want you to avoid your favorite starchy foods. Just rethink the ratios. You can have the pasta, but switch out some of the noodles for a tad more sauce. Have that piece of bread, but try eating it slowly with a generous amount of deep yellow, organic butter from pasture-fed cows. If you like stir-fry, don't just flavor your rice with it. Heap it on (making sure to use plenty of veggies) and cut back on the rice.

(87)
Rethink fast food.

When you're tempted to head for a fast food franchise because you're pressed for time and can't think of anything better, whip out your phone book and look up local restaurants, especially ethnic ones. You can get in and out of many of these about as fast as you could a national chain. If you have had bad experiences diving into uncharted waters in the past, then before you head out the door, see what others are saying; you can find reviews for practically any restaurant on the Internet. When we visit California, we seek out local Mexican eateries that feature plenty of the fresh produce California is famous for. On the East Coast, it makes more sense to look for good seafood, or a mom-and-pop pizza place that makes their dough from scratch and use olive oil and fresh garlic in their dressings and sauces. The point is, there's all kinds of satisfaction you'll never find if you habitually head for the golden arches.

(88)
Eat for your grandchildren's health.

We used to think genes never changed, that you inherited DNA from your parents, and pass on those genes to your children unaltered. We now know that our environment can influence our genes, directing the way they "express" themselves and even rewriting genetic information.

Genetic diseases are increasing, and the number of children with newly evolved minor chromosomal mutations associated with increased risk of autism, ADD, birth defects, and most other serious developmental disorders is much higher than experts predicted. This kind of chromosomal damage indicates unhealthy DNA and leads to abnormal physical growth. It is the fallout from decades of mindless eating. And it means that today, an average couple—both mom and dad—must take more care with their diet than in the past to have a healthy child.

(89)

If you can't get free-range, consider cutting your meat consumption.

You may have read that being vegetarian benefits your health. A large number of nutritionists, relying on data produced from a variety of studies, had been convinced that meat eaters are at higher than average risk for diabetes, cancer, and heart disease. But a recent study from Harvard's School of Public Health (by Dr. Renata Mecha) is shedding new light on those conclusions.

The older studies had failed to make the crucial distinction between processed and fresh. The Harvard study found that, contrary to popular belief, fresh meat consumption was not linked to a higher risk of these diseases. Only processed meat had this correlation.

But even this study failed to make a couple more key distinctions. Pasture-raised animals are higher in nutrients than grain-fed, and cooking method affects the ultimate nutrient content as well. I predict future studies that do recognize these distinctions will show that replacing overcooked feedlot meat with properly prepared meat from pastured animals can reduce your risk of heart attack, cancer, and diabetes from average to better than average.

Because certain nutrients can only be derived from animal products, it is crucial to find a source of healthy meat (this can include fish) if you have children or are planning a family.

(90)
Enjoy your salt.

The harms from using salt are vastly overstated. Salt is a naturally occurring mineral our bodies require for normal function. Salt makes vegetables taste better and facilitates their digestion. Salt does not cause hypertension. It does not cause weight gain. It does not elevate your risk of heart attack. In people with weak hearts and failing kidneys—who also have to restrict fluid intake, potassium, phosphate, and so on—yes, salt restriction is important. But salt doesn't cause heart failure or kidney damage, and if you don't have either condition, then you don't have to settle for unseasoned foods.

The real reason salt has a bad rap, as I see it, is that processed foods contain too many harmful compounds for doctors to keep track of—nitrates, oxidized fats, acrylamide, MSG, etc. But almost all processed foods also have added salt and taste noticeably salty. So, years ago, confronted by a bewildering array of ingredients in hot dogs, bacon-bits, cheese puffs, nacho chips and dips, and other junk foods that make people sick, doctors simply blamed the salt and, in spite of abundant research showing that *it's not the salt; it's the other stuff*, the salty association stuck. Patients also make the same mistake, blaming salt for their higher BP readings or swollen feet when all along it wasn't the salt, it was the salty-tasting junk.

Don't skip salt, skip the processed foods. Let your palate and good sense be your guide.

(91)
Limit caffeine to 2 cups a day.

Too much caffeine can irritate your GI tract and cause bloating, cramping, heartburn, diarrhea, and food intolerances. Caffeine's effect on your nerves can also create heartbeat irregularities and moodiness or irritability. And many caffeine addicts feel tired all the time.

As with alcohol, moderation is key. One or two cups of coffee or brewed tea is fine for most people, and both coffee and tea have been associated with health benefits, perhaps due to their antioxidant content. Avoid any drink to which caffeine has been added artificially, including power and energy drinks.

(92)
Replace soda with kombucha.

Soda is loaded with sugar, and the artificial sweeteners in diet sodas can have excitotoxic effects on your nerves and have been associated with a range of health problems. So what should you reach for to quench that hankering for refreshment?

Kombucha might suit ya. Kombucha is a naturally fermented, bubbly tea, often flavored with fruits and spices, that refreshes better than soda. Instead of a massive dose of sugar, you get an infusion of a variety of B vitamins and probiotics.

(93)
Make a dinner date with your whole family.

The Waltons did it. The Cunninghams did it. On the TV show Dallas, the Ewings did it too, even when the brothers were feudin'. In a perfect world, we'd all have time to sit down and eat dinner with our families every night. These days, that may not be realistic. So try this instead: Ask your kids to agree on a day of the week where everyone will sit down and eat a civilized dinner together. No computers. No Blackberries. No cell phones—and that means you, JR.

(94)

Don't be a tourist in your own town.

On a recent visit to Seattle, a friend recommended a hole-in-the-wall Filipino restaurant in the Pike's Place complex. As we took our seats at the counter, the man next to us—a chef at a local upscale restaurant (whose presence we took as a good omen)—suggested the house specialty, fish head soup. It was spectacular. When visiting UCLA, another friend directed us to a grocery store whose deli made delicious duck pâté from scratch. In San Francisco, a friend walked us to the sprawling Farmers Market in the Ferry Building where we loaded up on heirloom tomatoes, raw cheeses, artesanal olive oils, and fresh sourdough breads.

When your friends come to visit, treat them to the experience of stepping outside their comfort zone. Any tourist can grab a phone book and point to a national chain or eatery known as much for its decor as for its food. Rescue them from the world of boneless Buffalo wings, awesome extreme pepper jack pretzels, and red rocker margarita chicken poppers, and drag them to a sanctuary of authentic cuisine where strange and enticing aromas greet you at the door.

If you visit us here in Northern California, we'll take you to a place where the soup is made of lemongrass-scented beef broth with tripe and fishy meatballs. If you've never had *pho*, after leaving this restaurant, you will have a hard time believing that you had lived your entire life without ever once tasting Vietnam's national soup.

(95)

Don't fall for fake authentic.

When traveling, look for authentic local cuisine, not tourist trap cuisine posing as authentic. Cautious restaurant proprietors will shave the edges off of the region's true flavor—doing away with anything that might present the customer with a challenge to their palate—to make it seem more familiar to the traveler who is really just a tourist. Gradually the locals, who often depend on tourist dollars, lose touch with their culinary roots. I've met many young Hawaiians who had no idea that the *poi* (a mash of dried taro root reconstituted with water) their great-great-grandparents grew up on was typically eaten fermented, which gives the otherwise bland mush a real pungent flavor. This "deep end of the pool stuff," as travel TV host Andrew Zimmern calls such powerfully flavored cuisine, is often the first to be scratched off the menus of many larger chains and hotel restaurants.

(96)

Know that organic doesn't equal healthy.

You might shop where the air is so thick with patchouli incense that the smoke precipitates onto the ends of the cashier's dreadlocks. Still, this doesn't mean everything on the shelves is healthy. I shouldn't have to say this but experience has taught me otherwise: Organic cookies, sodas, and snack chips are not health foods. Nor are breakfast cereals, food bars, or trail mixes that taste like cookies. Even granola is mostly starch (empty calories), and most brands get their crunchiness by being baked in canola oil (as opposed to healthier coconut).

Organic standards have been softened as megastores continue to jump on the organic bandwagon, plying their political leverage to redefine the term. Organic is peachy, but today it makes more sense to include this labeling as one of the many things to consider when buying produce, or anything else. Sometimes the organic produce is so flabby, old, and tasteless, it's just not worth it. And sometimes, the manure used to fertilize organic spinach came from unhealthy cows (that aren't themselves raised well), and so your E. coli salad will put you in a coma. Some stores carry organic greens that have been shipped from thousands of miles away. By the time the veggies are flown, barged, trucked, and shelved, one pathogenic microbe with a doubling time of 20 minutes can become trillions. Additionally, many vitamins and antioxidants plummet shortly after the produce is picked. Buy fresh and local when possible and let your taste buds—not just the word "organic"—do the talking.

(97)
Entertain.

Luke and I are just not Martha Stewart-y enough to have known that the secret to successful dinner parties is preparing ahead. We've served undercooked steaks, burnt homemade pizzas, and soggy stir fries. Because they have to be made on the spot and one mistimed step can ruin everything, these were destined to be disasters from the get-go. We had to learn the hard way that the best foods for entertaining are those that can sit and rest in a slow cooker or Dutch oven, where extra time doesn't make much of a difference. A large roast, braised meats, and soups and stews (chili is always a winner) are examples of dishes that help make entertaining friends more entertaining for you.

Doctor's Orders

Michael Pollan talks about the notional tomato, "the *idea* of a tomato, but flavorless" and not as healthy for us. In many ways, we have bought into the idea of notional health. We are so busy watching cholesterol and blood pressure numbers, we aren't paying attention to the fact that our minds and bodies are degenerating more rapidly than normal. I suggest we redirect our focus away from "risk factors" and pay more attention to what we eat, where our food comes from, and how we cook it. Risk factors are useful to you only in that they provide feedback that can help gauge how successfully you are providing your body with the right nutrients. I find the most valuable risk factors to be those that gauge inflammation, and I will discuss them here.

More health practitioners are coming to appreciate the role of diet in controlling inflammation and regaining health. Following the Rules outlined in Parts I, II, and III, and getting off the pro-inflammatory Western diet, are key to tapping in to your body's amazing capacity for regeneration. But there is more to health than getting off the Western diet. In order for your body to put all that good food to use rebuilding more functional tissues and cells, you need to send the right kinds of regenerative signals. To facilitate optimal growth and body functioning at every age you need proper exercise, sleep, and to be free of drugs that will interfere with cellular processes. In this section, I help you recognize your real risk factors, and outline a simple set of instructions that have helped my patients achieve weight loss, improve bone density, avoid recurring infections, and so much more.

(1)
Know your risk for diabetes.

The old thinking on diabetes—and, unfortunately, what most people still hear—is that when the insulin-making "beta" cells in your pancreas are overworked by a high-sugar diet, they poop out, and your blood sugar rises. Now we know better. It's not just sugary foods; you can avoid all sugars and still get diabetes. The number one cause of diabetes is a pro-inflammatory diet. I've listed this Doctor's Order first because, on a pro-inflammatory diet, every kind of cell in your body may develop some level of abnormal function long before your pancreas poops out. The point is: *The same body-wide cell damage that leads eventually to diabetes puts you at higher risk for almost every other illness in the books.*

Don't wait for high blood sugar levels to develop before taking action. If you eat junk for meals, are overweight, have high blood pressure, high triglycerides, a high LDL to HDL cholesterol ratio, or don't exercise, then you already have cell damage and are likely on your way to developing diabetes. And once you have clinically obvious diabetes, your tendons and joints may be damaged to the point that exercise is painful, thus trapping you in a cycle of weight gain and physical deterioration.

To break out of that cycle, you need to return your body to health at a cellular level.

A cell is kind of like a hotel with a doorman at each of its entry and exit portals to regulate the flow of chemicals into and out of the cell. A bad diet combined with no exercise makes that doorman sleepy and sloppy, so the cell doors that allow sugar, for instance, to go inside don't open fast enough when insulin signals that blood sugar is heading upward. When sluggish portals delaying the flow of sugar traffic into the cell, inside, your cell is starving for energy, while outside the lines of glucose molecules waiting to get into Hotel Cell are winding around the block—and your blood sugar rises too high. The cell also has little doors for minerals, vitamins, amino acids, and more, and all the little doormen must stay alert for each of these chemicals to keep all your cells operating smoothly.

If you have inflammation-damage affecting your cells, your tissues may become less receptive to *any* hormone, not just to insulin, so early signs of diabetes include multiple hormonal problems. In men, testosterone insensitivity causes ED, and in women, estrogen insensitivity causes menstrual irregularities and infertility. As inflammation continues and cellular injury spreads, the cascade of damage extending outward from one disrupted system can eventually grow to affect many others, which is why diabetes has been associated with every medical problem in the book, from osteoporosis to lupus to Alzheimer's to cancer.

I tell my patients that medications won't reverse diabetes because medications don't reverse membrane damage; only good diet can do that. Though medications bring blood sugar down, the sugar goes into fat cells, so a common side effect is weight gain. My highest priority in treating diabetes—even in its earliest, preclinical stage—is getting you on a better diet.

The good news of course is once you get your diet on track, your body will bounce back strong, and your risk of all other illnesses will plummet.

(2)
Rethink cancer.

The war on cancer will not be won with technology. Consider this: Four out of five early invasive breast cancers detected on mammograms may disappear in time without surgery, radiation, or chemo, according to Norway's public health statistician Dr. Per-Henrich Zahl. This may sound shocking but you probably have cancer cells in your body right now. Autopsy studies find prostate cancer in one of ten men in their 20s, and breast cancer in four of ten women in their 40s. If cancer were universally deadly, few of us would make it past 50. So something must be protecting us.

There is. It's called "immune surveillance," a process in which your white blood cells recognize and destroy malignancies without you ever being aware of a problem. This is not some fringe, new age philosophy; Yale University's Dr. R. J. Papac tells us that "Spontaneous regression of cancer is reported in virtually all types of human cancer." Far from being a universal death sentence, cancer seems something our bodies can defeat—provided our immune systems are healthy.

To avoid succumbing to cancer, I advise my patients to fortify their immune-system army with an anti-cancer shield, one made of nourishing foods, exercise, and sleep. It's also vital you keep your body free of inflammation, which distracts and disarms white blood cells. Stress, sedentary life, overeating, smoking, excessive alcohol consumption, and foods containing toxic oils and sugar all cause inflammation, opening the door to malignancies. Swing that door open often enough, and one just might slip through and take root.

(3)

Get your blood sugar level checked.

Fasting blood sugar says more about your overall health than any other blood test, including your cholesterol level. Current guidelines define normal fasting glucose as under 100. But many medical specialists believe this is too high, and that under 90 might be a better cutoff point. I agree with this stricter definition of "normal" because, in my experience, people with fasting glucoses higher than 89 are already experiencing problems associated with diabetes. Most strikingly, above that threshold of 89 a person suddenly becomes much more likely to suffer a heart attack or stroke.

According to our current standard of care, a doctor shouldn't diagnose diabetes until the patient has fasting blood sugar levels over 125. In my opinion, waiting that long is dangerous. Typically, patients with fasting sugar levels of 90 or higher already have hidden atherosclerosis and more obvious problems like weight gain, high blood pressure, erectile dysfunction, hormonal problems, low "good" cholesterol, high "bad" cholesterol, allergic problems, and stiff and achy joints. By the time fasting sugar climbs to 125, serious medical problems like heart attack, heart failure, stroke, kidney and nerve damage, and uncontrolled weight gain are very common.

As a cautionary note, in my nearly 20 years in medicine, every patient I've met who developed cancer at an early age had a major sweet tooth. If you have a sweet tooth, or if your fasting blood sugar level is 90 or higher and you want to get back to normal, following the rules in this book will help wean you away from sweets and bring those numbers down.

(4)
Know what your cholesterol numbers *really* mean.

It is commonly said that women have fewer heart attacks because we have more HDL, and HDL is "good." This is only partly true. Women do have fewer heart attacks, and more HDL. *But HDL is not what's keeping our arteries clean.* Besides, this idea that HDL protects a woman's arteries still leaves us with the question: *Why do women have higher HDL?*

For men and women both, understanding HDL is key to understanding *if* your high cholesterol is a problem. To understand why high cholesterol is not always a problem, and what all your numbers mean, let's back up and take a look at the bigger picture, one that includes the whole body, and both sexes.

Let's start with a typical cholesterol test report, which has four numbers: Total cholesterol, HDL ("good" cholesterol), LDL ("bad" cholesterol), and triglycerides. All four refer to the fact that cholesterol and dietary fats flow through your blood vessels inside particles called *lipoproteins*, which have different densities. The number one job of all lipoproteins is to deliver their payload of triglycerides, fat-soluble vitamins, and other nutriment (choline, phospholipids, etc.) to your brain, muscles, skin, and everywhere else. When that delivery process breaks down, your cholesterol numbers go out of whack and your arteries can get caked up with the fat and protein breakdown products of undeliverable lipoprotein particles.

Here's how that caking-up starts:

The liver makes LDL from the triglycerides and other fats you eat, and when the fats in your diet are pro-inflammatory (trans fats, for instance), the liver puts those bad fats into your LDL particles, too. *But the bad fats change how the LDL particle works.* Particles containing pro-inflammatory fat can't get delivered into tissues like they should. So on a bad diet, there are simply more LDL particles in your bloodstream at any one time, which raises LDL and/or triglyceride levels (which one goes up how high also depends on your sugar intake and other factors). Trapped and recirculating in your bloodstream far longer than they should be, the particles eventually "spoil," oxidizing and melting into a toxic sludge that deposits on the delicate inner lining of your arteries, inflaming them and leading to atherosclerosis.

Meanwhile, what's a person's pro-inflammatory diet doing to their HDL? HDL is not made by the liver. Instead, HDL is made primarily in the fat under our skin and contains many fats that were delivered to the skin by LDL. But if the fats in LDL particles don't get delivered into the skin, the skin can't make as much HDL, and HDL levels go down. Another reason HDL drops has to do with the fact that sugar destroys the proteins by which laboratories identify HDL. With identifying proteins destroyed, HDL appears to drop, though the particles remain in circulation and, like LDL, they too eventually "spoil" and become arterial toxic-sludge build-up.

Next, I'll talk about the male-female differences. A big reason a woman can make more HDL than a man who is eating the same foods stems from the fact that women have more fat under our skin than men. *But higher HDL is not the biggest factor keeping a woman's arteries clean.* The single most important circumstance protecting women's arteries appears to be the fact that menstruation keeps women's iron levels relatively low. Iron can oxidize certain fats and this directly damages LDL and HDL particles. The relatively high iron levels in a man's bloodstream makes his lipoproteins oxidize, or "spoil," faster, damaging his arteries at a faster rate than a woman's. Things even out a few decades after menopause, when a woman's iron levels become more similar to a man's.

The following paragraphs describe how I interpret your cholesterol numbers and what I advise my patients to do. (For references, I refer the interested reader to *Deep Nutrition*, which cites the research data supporting these statements.)

LDL should be less than three times HDL.

If you HDL is 50, your LDL should be 150 or lower. A ratio of three to one is okay, but a ratio of two to one is better. An out-of-whack ratio indicates damaged LDL particles may be building up in your arteries. You can improve your ratio with exercise, adding fresh vegetables (not fruits) to your diet, making sure not to overcook red meat (the iron in red meat damages fats in your food just as it does in the bloodstream), and eliminating vegetable oils.

Triglycerides should be 70 to 150.

Triglycerides over 150 come from eating vegetable oils and too much sugar. The most common sources of vegetable oils are fried foods from restaurants, pre-made salad dressings, snack chips, granola bars, pastries, muffins, cookies, and microwavable meals. The most common sources of excessive sugar come from soda, a high-carb diet, and excessive fruit and juice consumption.

HDL should be over 45 in men and over 55 in women.

See the next Doctor's Order.

(5)
Get your HDL numbers up.

In 2010, at a symposium entitled "When low cholesterol isn't enough," leading cardiologists acknowledged that low HDL is more dangerous than high LDL. If your HDL is low (under 40) and you get it up to 60 naturally—without medications—you melt your risk of heart attack to half (men) or a quarter (women) of what it was. Proportional LDL reduction does not have such an effect.

Eight ways to raise your HDL naturally:

- Reduce intake of processed or overcooked meats
- Cut dietary sugar and starch
- Swap vegetable oils for natural fats
- Increase fresh vegetable consumption
- Increase dietary garlic and other herbs and spices
- Increase total daily sleep
- Increase level of exercise
- Quit smoking

Low HDL can be caused by smoking, stress, and lack of sleep or exercise. But for most of my patients, the cause is related to diabetes which, in turn, is related to unhealthy lifestyle and dietary choices (see Doctor's Order number One). Bad diet, smoking, and lack of exercise combine to leave your lipoproteins highly vulnerable to the spoiling effects of oxidation that make HDL numbers drop and LDL rise. So what do you do? Eat healthy fats along with plenty of antioxidants to rehabilitate your metabolism and keep your lipoprotein particles fresh and circulating normally.

(6)
Forget the idea that saturated fat and cholesterol are bad for you.

A lot of people have been convinced that cholesterol builds up inside arteries like sludge in a pipe, squeezing off blood supply more and more until one day—*boom!*—you get a heart attack or stroke. The best science points to another way of thinking about cholesterol.

If you scrape your skin badly, a scab forms. The scab is comprised mostly of protein. If your artery is damaged by accumulated pro-inflammatory fats (from deposits of undeliverable lipoprotein particles), the body responds by creating another kind of scab, an atherosclerotic plaque, a kind of patch which seals, strengthens, and waterproofs the damaged section of arterial wall. This "scab" contains protein, calcium, and *cholesterol*. Once formed, arterial plaques effectively reinforce the weakened artery and, provided the inflammation does not continue, can remain stable for a lifetime. Telling you that you can prevent the formation of these plaques by avoiding cholesterol-rich foods makes as little sense as telling you that you can prevent skin scabs by avoiding protein-rich foods.

Cholesterol-containing arterial plaques are your body's response to arterial damage, not the cause. The way to prevent arterial damage, and prevent heart attacks and strokes, is to avoid foods that destabilize your lipoproteins and otherwise lead to arterial inflammation. And how do you do that? By following all the rules in this book. Far from being your mortal enemy, saturated fat and cholesterol are vital elements of a healthy diet.

Here are a few reasons why:

Seven benefits of dietary saturated fat and cholesterol:

- Cholesterol-rich foods are typically loaded with other nutrients
- Both cholesterol and saturated fats suppress appetite, which can prevent overeating
- Increasing saturated fat and cholesterol can raise your HDL ("good" cholesterol)
- Saturated fats prevent inflammation by protecting other nutrients in your food from oxidative damage
- Saturated fats prevent inflammation by protecting cell membranes and lipoproteins from free radical damage
- There is no traditional diet that does not contain foods rich in animal fat
- Saturated fats and cholesterol help you absorb fat-soluble nutrients such as:

  Essential fatty acids omega-3 and -6

  Vitamin A

  Vitamin D

  Vitamin E

  Vitamin K

  Most phytonutrients

  Most antioxidants

  Brain- and muscle-building compounds such as lecithin, biotin, and choline.

(7)
Get your vitamin D level checked.

Nearly 80 percent of Americans are vitamin D deficient by mid-winter, according to some studies, and the numbers aren't much better in summer. That's concerning because vitamin D is crucial to normal functioning of numerous body tissues, most famously bone, nerve, and the immune system. Low vitamin D seems to accelerate age-related degeneration and inflammatory illnesses (inflammatory illnesses include everything from arthritis and allergies to cancer and lupus). It seems that every time researchers study a given disease, they find it is more likely to occur in people who lack adequate D. That's why I strongly recommend you get your levels checked.

If your level is significantly below 30 ng/ml, you may need to supplement, at least in the short term, with an artificially synthesized form of vitamin D called ergosterol, or D_2, which is available in 50,000 i.u. tablets. If you are not severely deficient, I recommend at least 2000 i.u. of D_3. Once your levels are back to normal, you may be able to keep them there with naturally occurring D from animal foods or sunlight.

Best food sources of vitamin D

- Liver (and liver oils)
- Blood (i.e., blood sausage, or *bodin noir*)
- Kidneys (look for recipes online)
- Egg yolks

These must come from animals that have had access to sun, or their tissues, eggs, etc. are unlikely to have adequate D. To find them, you may have to do some web surfing and some legwork. I recommend going to your local farmer's markets and asking around, looking up butcher shops or slaughterhouses (some are listed under the term *abattoir*) in the yellow pages, and checking out the very helpful website EatWild.com, which has a nationwide database of pasture-based farms.

Keep in mind, pasteurized milk is fortified with D_3, but cheese, yoghurt, raw milk, and dairy products other than pasteurized milk are not, and are poor sources of D.

Many mushrooms make ergosterol (D_2), which has similar but not identical effects compared to vitamin D_3, and some believe there is a risk of calcium ending up in tissues where it doesn't belong when D_2 is used in place of D_3.

Sensible UV Exposure:

If you stay in the sun too long, the continued UV exposure starts destroying vitamin D—and your skin. Your skin tells you if you stayed too long by turning red. Unfortunately, at that point it's too late. So pay attention to how long it took for you to tan or redden for next time.

Most of us can make D in our skin, but the ability to do so diminishes after age 40. For a young person, 20 minutes of full-body exposure to summer sun (wearing a bikini or swim trunks, no more than 10 minutes per side) between 10 AM and 2 PM provides around 20,000 i.u. If you wear shorts and a T-shirt, you should aim to get 20 minutes of sun three days a week. You can make D at other times of the year as well. For details appropriate to your latitude and season check out Dr. Michael Holick's web site: http://www.vitamindhealth.org

(8)

Be wary of cholesterol-lowering medication.

When your doctor says he wants to put you on a cholesterol-lowering drug, the presumption is you'll live longer on the drug than off of it. It's satisfying, the idea that by simply taking a daily pill you are proactively combating heart disease and stroke. The problem is, though the pills lower cholesterol successfully, unless you fall within a very specific patient demographic, these drugs will not, in reality, help you live longer. In fact, they very well may hasten your death. However, since more and more insurance companies are financially penalizing physicians who do not put everyone with an LDL over 100-130 on a cholesterol pill, doctors are incentivized against telling you about side effects of these drugs.

There are three kinds of drugs that lower cholesterol. Repeated studies comparing two of the three kinds of drugs to placebo pills (sugar pills) show that the people taking the placebo live longer. These two classes are fibrates and cholesterol-resorbtion inhibitors (Tricor, Vytorin, and Zetia are examples). I don't prescribe them. The third kind of cholesterol-lowering drug is the most popular, called statins. Studies show that statins do prevent heart attacks and strokes in carefully selected groups of people, but most of these trials are drug-company funded and of questionable reliability—and even here the evidence that statins prolong life is limited, at best.

Statins block an enzyme called HMGCoA-reductase, which your body uses to produce cholesterol and many other metabolic products that your organs need to function normally. Side effects include, but are not limited to, memory problems, infections, fatigue, depression, dizziness, muscle pain, and muscle weakness. This last one is of particular concern to patients suffering from heart failure, which is essentially a weakening of heart muscle. The evidence against statin use in heart-failure patients is clear, yet practitioners seem afraid to advise their heart-failure patients to discontinue them (something I'd like to see change). Statins can also cause or worsen diabetes, and diabetes is the leading cause of heart attack and stroke, so giving statins to diabetics—or anyone with high blood sugar—seems to me a rather illogical practice.

In my experience, many statin side effects are severe enough to affect quality of life. But because few physicians are properly educated about statins, they mistakenly believe any harms of these medications can be detected in a blood test. I frequently see people who are suffering from what could be statin side effects, such as tendonitis, depression, vertigo, or dementia, which the prescribing doctor has typically attributed to excessive activity, stress, inner ear diseases, or aging. When I see such ongoing symptoms in patients on statins, I feel obligated to inform them that stopping statins might help.

Statins are now so widely used we're treating them almost like a vitamin pill, and I've heard more than one colleague suggest they should be put in the municipal water supply. I think this cavalier attitude is dangerous. Statins are powerful drugs whose use is medically justified in a very select group of patients. I prescribe them primarily to male smokers who have no heart failure, no history of cancer, and who have already had a heart attack or stroke and continue to smoke.

(9)
Be wary of bone-density pills.

One of the most popular brands of bone density drugs claims to "work with your body" to help stop and reverse bone loss. In reality, such drugs (called bisphosphonates) don't work with your body at all.

Few people realize that bone density drugs are officially approved only for women with either a prior osteoporotic fracture or a bone-density *T-score* less than negative two. Yet I see patients on these drugs who don't even meet the official qualifications. Even if you do, the drugs will not reduce your risk of fracture as effectively as *proper* (see next page) supplementation. The drugs reduce your fracture risk by thirty percent, and proper supplementation reduces your risk by fifty percent.

If you already supplement and want to start taking the drugs, you should know that combining drugs and supplementation won't help because of the way the drugs work. Bone is a living tissue that is constantly undergoing a process called *remodeling*, wherein old sections of bone are reabsorbed so that new, healthier bone can be rebuilt. The drugs interfere with the remodeling process, the process by which bones regenerate, by blocking your body's ability to reabsorb the calcium from old, worn-out sections of bone. When calcium sticks around longer, bones appear denser, which we have been fooled into equating with healthy bone. (A piece of chalk also appears very dense on an X-Ray.) Unfortunately, blocking the remodeling process can, over time, weaken bones severely. There have been cases in which people on these drugs have developed jawbone necrosis after dental work, or were just walking along when their thighbones snapped underneath them. These terrible side effects have prompted those who study bone density drugs to call for limiting their use. I no longer prescribe them. Unfortunately, as long as the media still run misleading advertisements, the use of these dangerous medications will continue.

The following builds strong, healthy bones:

- Weightlifting exercise three times a week (sends the signals for bones to grow stronger)
- Bone stocks twice a week (reverses aging by rebuilding joints and bone matrix, see Rule 48)
- Three daily servings of either dairy products, bone-in fish like mackerel or sardines, or dark green leafy vegetables like collards and kale (for minerals and vitamin K) or supplemental daily Calcium 500 to 1000 mg with Magnesium 250 mg and Zinc 100% RDA
- Sunshine for 20 minutes three days a week, or supplemental vitamin D_3, 2000 I.U. per day
- If you take calcium supplements, you must take supplemental D_3—calcium alone can cause heart disease and bone spurs. For this reason and more, I prefer people skip calcium supplements in favor of calcium-rich foods

I promised myself I wouldn't clutter this book with footnotes because *Deep Nutrition* contains the supporting science. But I'm making a number of controversial claims here that were not discussed in *Deep Nutrition*, and feel that references are in order.[1]

---

1 BMJ 2010;340:b5463, Sports Med 2005; 35 (9): 779-830, Altern Med Rev. 2008 Mar;13(1):21-33, Am Fam Physician. 2008 Sep 1;78(5):579-581

(10)
Take pain seriously.

Pain may be a warning from your body that something you're doing needs to change. In my experience, the problem is usually too much sugar, too much protein, inadequate sleep, and ineffective or no exercise.

Cutting back on activity is not the answer. In another Doctor's Order, I go into more detail about why your body needs exercise just to function. But for now, suffice it to say that after many years of active practice, I've seen the combination of extra sleep, cutting sugar, adding bone broths with protein-rich foods, and healthy exercise act as a miracle cure for those patients suffering from chronic pain.

Don't put off addressing chronic pain issues. If you don't make these changes, your discomfort may grow to the point that you are in too much pain to exercise or work.

(11)
Rethink heartburn.

If you can't eat food without feeling pain, then something is seriously wrong—even if your test results come out normal. It may only be that you are eating too much. Or, it may be that your stomach lining is inflamed by vegetable oils and oxidized fats. It's also possible that you may be extra sensitive to caffeine and the other potentially irritating compounds in coffee and tea.

Don't accept that you need to stay on antacid pills for life; long-term use has been associated with low bone density and other health problems. Start by cutting out vegetable oils, cutting down on caffeine, and adding a few probiotic-containing foods to your weekly regimen (or daily probiotic supplements), and your system should start to heal. Make sure to follow the rules on combining food discussed earlier in this book. Ask your doctor if she is familiar with "leaky gut," a term alternative practitioners use to describe what I would call mild-but-generalized intestinal inflammation. If your doctor is not familiar with the root causes of intestinal inflammation and you've already seen the appropriate medical specialists, then working with a naturopath on this may be your best course of action.

(12)

Rethink arthritis.

If you are an athlete who depends on good joint health, you need to do three things for your joints: get sleep, avoid pro-inflammatory vegetable oils and sugar, and eat bone broths with protein-rich foods. I've already talked about how "bad" protein damages collagen (Rule 57) and broth replenishes it, and I will address the other three recommendations here.

Let's talk about sleep first. Normal daytime activity traumatizes the collagen fibrils in your muscles, tendons, and joints. At night, as you sleep, these tissues swell slightly as your body makes repairs. If you feel stiff when you wake in the morning, it indicates that you haven't given this healing process enough time. If you fail to get adequate sleep for days or weeks on end, you are setting yourself up for potentially mobility-limiting aches and pains.

Next, let's talk about vegetable oil. The fatty acids in vegetable oils can inflame your tissues, especially on a low-nutrient diet. Inflammation can activate collagen-destroying enzymes called *collagenases*. These enzymes are normally triggered by bacterial infection. Bad diets (and stress) can activate collagenases in the wrong places at the wrong times. This gradually weakens your connective tissues so that your joints are easily injured.

Finally, sugar. Sugar accelerates wear and tear by acting as a corrosive in your joints. Sugar binds with proteins in the connective tissue from which your moving parts are constructed, and any motion in a joint that's loaded up with sugar can grind away at the collagen, leading to snapping, cracking, popping, stiff, achy joints.

(13)

Rethink headaches.

If you suffer from frequent headaches, your doctor has probably already recommended cutting artificial sweeteners, MSG, sulfate-containing red wines, limiting caffeine, and reducing stress. If you've tried all that (and more serious causes of headache have been ruled out) then try cutting your sugar and carbs.

Carb-rich diets cause headaches because they cause hormone level fluctuations. When blood sugar starts to rise, your body releases insulin and other hormones to reduce it. When blood sugar falls, adrenaline and other hormones bring it back up. On a high-carb or sugary diet, your body is forced to release all those different sets of hormones much more often than when you're on a low-carb and low-sugar diet. As hormone levels rise and fall, the fluctuations have subtly irritating effects on your nervous system. Top that off with regular infusions of caffeine or analgesic medication, inadequate restorative sleep, and a stressful lifestyle, and you have a recipe for neural inflammation and headaches.

I'm not going to tell you that cutting sugar and carbs eliminates headaches in all people. But even those patients with the worst headaches often experience significant relief simply by making this dietary change.

(14)
Avoid antibacterial soaps.

People are buying these soaps gallons at a time because they hope to make their homes more safe and sanitary. Unfortunately, regular use may actually make a home more dangerous.

Most of us have heard about "drug resistant superbugs." The evolution of superbugs in your body works like this. Let's say you have a sinus infection and take amoxicillin. If any of the infectious bacteria have some strategy by which they can evade the effects of the antibiotic, then they will go on to reproduce new generations of bacteria that are likewise resistant. This is how "superbugs" are bred.

These new antibacterial soaps encourage a similar evolution in your sinks, on your countertops, on your skin—wherever you use them. Scientists theorize we are seeing an emergence of bacteria that produce collagen-penetrating enzymes to burrow beneath the surface of our skin, escaping contact with antibacterial skin products and surviving. Such burrowing bacteria can also enter a tiny cut on your child's leg and then rapidly abscess, or even progress to gangrene. What's more, the antibiotic-resistant superbugs are now very common, but are typically kept in check by "good bacteria" on our skin. Antibacterial soaps can wipe out these good guys. The patients I've seen with serious superbug infections have also used antibacterial soaps or had been in close contact with someone who did.

Avoid antibiotic, antimicrobial, or antibacterial agents in soaps and lotions. The most common agent is triclosan.

(15)

Don't expect most supplements to do very much.

Though compelling advertising claims can persuade us to believe supplements are powerful natural cures, the reality is something else entirely. Supplements are processed for extended shelf life, and just as with all processed foods, much of the original nutritional value is lost in the journey through the factory. The processing is especially damaging to memory and brain supplements.

What's more, many people who supplement in an attempt to make up for nutrient deficiencies don't get what they're missing from the supplements. We need lots of different kinds of nutrients, so the probability that the collection of chemicals a person happens to pull off the shelves will happen to fill the void in their dietary regimen is vanishingly small. If you're thinking, *at least they can't hurt me*, that may only be partially true; man-made vitamins are not identical to the real thing and may contain harmful vitamin-mimics.

Supplements can, however, help make up for the depletion of soil minerals and the fact that—let's face it—unless you grew up eating them, organ meats are not easy to work into your diet.

I recommend these supplements:

- Magnesium 250 mg
- Vitamin D, 2000 i.u., especially in winter
- Fish or cod liver oil for long-chain omega-3 fats during childhood. Flax oil for short-chain omega-3 after age 18. (Children can't elongate omega-3, but adults can.)

(16)
Exercise—just do it.

If exercise could somehow be converted into pill form it would be considered the miracle drug of the century. Vigorous exercise reduces every marker of inflammation we can measure. It has been shown to be at least as effective at treating depression as any anti-depressant on the market. Exercise cuts an Alzheimer's patient's risk of institutionalization in half. And one study showed post-menopausal women who exercised for six months regained lost height from some areas of their spine.[2]

Failing to exercise sends a powerful signal to every tissue in your body to atrophy. So why don't more people do it?

Maybe there's the perception that exercise is something to do only when you want to lose weight. Or people presume their aches and pains will get worse if they exercise. (Lack of exercise is actually one of the most common causes of back, neck, and hip pain.) Of course, there are a number of legitimate medical conditions that prevent people from exercising as much as they'd like. But no matter what your present health condition, you should exercise as much as you are able while you are able. I'm not exaggerating when I tell you that just about every last one of my patients who exercises regularly is healthy, and almost every last patient who neglects exercise is not.

---

[2] A 6-mo home-based exercise program may slow vertebral height loss. J Clin Densitom. 2003 Winter;6(4):391-400

(17)
Do yoga before breakfast.

The ancient Chinese discipline of Qigong holds that morning stretching is necessary for the flow of vital chi, and a prerequisite for good health. Professional athletes now take stretching, and yoga in particular, as seriously as they do cardio and strength training. In my experience, few patients who have been introduced to the benefits of yoga ever give it up.

Over the age of forty, a few minutes of balance exercises every morning can help prevent falls and broken bones. There's also evidence that regular stretching can prevent, or at least delay, repetitive motion injury. You know you are stretching correctly when it feels good. Done right, you can feel like someone just gave you a nice massage.

(18)
Get your heart rate up.

A lot of people believe they're getting aerobic exercise when they clean up around the house or go strolling for bargains around the mall. Housework and strolling are good things, but they're not going to give you the benefits of a real workout.

Aerobic exercise, or cardio, that increases your heart rate includes activities like biking, swimming, jogging, and uphill or brisk walking. I'm talking about working out till you breathe hard, break a sweat, and your heart rate kicks up to the aerobic zone for your age. (Establish this with your doctor.)

Done properly, aerobic exercise is a great way to "clean your system." It reduces all kinds of inflammatory chemicals and will improve your HDL and blood sugar levels, while keeping your heart, lungs, and circulatory system in good shape. Real exercise releases all sorts of growth factors and mood-elevating opioids, and when combined with a healthy diet, exercise has been shown to trigger regeneration of every tissue of the body (see next Doctor's Order).

(19)
Exercise anaerobically.

Think weightlifting, or chopping wood. Think focus and intense concentration. Think no pain, no gain, because real anaerobic exercise involves pushing yourself.

The word means, literally, without oxygen. During anaerobic exercise you are pushing your body hard enough that your blood can't replenish the exercising tissues with oxygen, and they simply run out. This creates the classic burning in your muscles, which means you are going to feel a little sore tomorrow. That soreness also signals your body to build more muscle, and when it goes away you'll be transformed.

If aerobic exercise is about cleaning out your system, anaerobic exercise is about building it bigger, stronger, and faster. Studies show that weightlifting, for example, expands not just muscle mass, but also the tendons and bone that work with the muscle as a unit. It also improves coordination, making you faster, and improves memory, stimulating the growth of new brain cells *at any age*—a feat once thought impossible.

(20)
Learn to dance.

If you feel as if you might be allergic to exercise, then trick your body into action by doing workouts that are way too fun. Try a Zumba class, or ballroom, folk, or contra dancing. Classes are usually inexpensive or free at neighborhood centers, churches, and your local schools. (Craigslist is a good resource, too.)

(21)
Sleep.

If you think you don't have time to sleep, think again. Studies show that people who push themselves and keep their usual work schedule when they feel an illness coming on actually miss more work than people who stay home early to nip their infection in the bud.

Sleep is a key element missing from many people's weight loss programs. Research also tells us that sleep is key to growth (especially important in childhood), memory function, immune system health, and treating diabetes. While we sleep, our bodies are very busy. At night, our brain cells record the day's experiences into memory, cells called *fibroblasts* manufacture collagen required for bone and joint health, immune system cells pump out cancer- and infection fighting chemicals—and that's just the beginning. Chronic sleep deprivation creates real, physiologic stress that breaks our bodies down and can be measured using blood markers of systemic inflammation. In *Stroke of Insight*, neuroanatomist and author Jill Bolte Taylor says that the biggest lesson she took from the experience of having and recovering from a stroke was the importance of restorative sleep. If you're sick, even with something minor like a cold, you need extra sleep to get over your infection faster and get back to work.

Appendix A

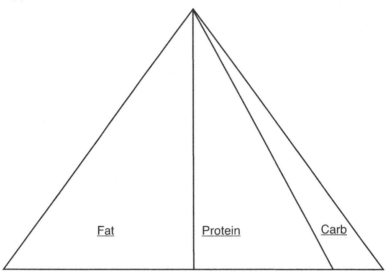

Fat · Protein · Carb

Sweets

Starches
0-3 daily
potatoes
pasta
grains
legumes

Animal foods
2-4 daily servings
(a variety, including eggs,
dairy, fish, fowl, pork, and
grazing animals, to include as
many tissue types as possible)

Vegetables (and Fruits)
5-6 daily servings
fermented (3-4 per week)
gently cooked (2-4 per day), fresh (2-4 per day)
For each serving of fruit, eat 3 servings of veggies

Appendix A

The Traditional Diet Pyramid

The top pyramid is a rough guide to general food categories. The point is not to memorize exact percentages. The take-home point is, don't fear fat. Roughly half of your daily calories should come from healthy fats. This is because fat enhances the bioavailability and nutrient transport of fat-soluble vitamins while suppressing appetite and keeping you from overdosing on volume (especially important for starchy foods and meats). Saturated fats should compose roughly half of your total fat intake. Together with cholesterol, saturated fat facilitates digestion and appetite control. Your intestinal cells require saturated fat and cholesterol to manufacture the chylomicrons into which most dietary fats must be incorporated to be absorbed, including essential fatty acids omega-3 and -6, vitamins A, D, E, and K, biotin, choline, brain-building phospholipids, and the flavinoids and lipid antioxidants in plant foods.

The bottom pyramid is your guide to traditional food portioning.

Vegetables form the foundation of the traditional food pyramid diagrammed here because, for most people today, it is easier to find high-quality fresh vegetables than animal products. If you live in an area where high-quality and pasture-raised meat, eggs, and fresh dairy are more readily available than high-quality and fresh vegetables, then these products (when prepared according to traditional methods and when dairy is consumed raw) may form the foundation of your diet instead.

Animal foods must come from healthy sources and must be prepared so as to protect their nutritional value. Cooked red meats, poultry, and pork should be consumed with bone broths at least half of the time. Dairy, eggs, and fish may safely be consumed raw, but I

155

encourage this practice only when high-quality sources are available to you fresh.

Grains and legumes are best when sprouted first, as this reduces antinutrients and awakens enzymes that convert starch to more complex nutrients.

Fruit products (jam, juice), chocolate, and homemade baked goods (with butter or coconut oil) or ice cream should be occasional treats. Desserts should be enjoyed twice a week at most.

First Steps:

To ease your way into this program, start with breakfast. By switching out boxed cereals, frozen waffles, instant oatmeals, and donuts, and by following the menu suggestions on page 163, you'll be setting your taste buds and your insulin levels on course for a healthier day.

Appendix B

Healthy Shopping List

Dried goods and pantry items
White flour, preferably organic unbleached
Wheat berries
Barley
Oats, or oat-groats
Dried beans: kidney, black, garbanzo, pinto, etc.
Granulated sugar
Sea salt
Garlic
Onions
Shallots
Dried mushrooms

Dried fruits and fruit products
Raisins, especially yellow raisins
Cranberries
Currants
Apricots
Mango
Papaya
Shredded coconut
Unsweetened juices (sparingly, fruits are healthier)

Starchy foods
Pasta, especially organic or heirloom (gentle drying techniques)
Jasmine rice
Brown rice (be aware that this doesn't keep as well as white)
Sprouted grain breads and English muffins, including cinnamon raisin
Sourdough breads

Potatoes, preferably organic and not Russet (clones bred for fast food French fries)
White corn tortillas (be sure to select the soft type with no oils)
Sprouted grain tortillas
Granola made with coconut oil (health food stores often carry one or two bins of this)
Pretzels (oil-free)
Crackers made with no oil or approved oils (see Rule 3)
Bagel chips (without vegetable oils)

Nuts and seeds
(For all nuts and seeds, raw or sprouted are better than dry roasted. Avoid nuts roasted in vegetable oil. Soaking and then roasting nuts is not necessary unless you find it aids digestion.)
Almonds
Brazil nuts (excellent sources of Magnesium and Selenium)
Cashews
Walnuts (excellent sources of omega-3, which is damaged by roasting)
Pecans
Peanuts, in shell are freshest
Pine nuts
Pumpkin seeds
Sunflower seeds
Peanut and nut butters made without added sugars (best when ground fresh at your local health food store!)

157

Appendix B

Tip for seasonings and spices: Grind your own when possible, especially pepper, cardamom seed, nutmeg, and mustard seed

Cooking oils, sauces, and pantry items
Olive oil
Peanut oil
Balsamic vinegar
White vinegar
Fish sauce (Squid brand is naturally brewed)
Oyster sauce (look for "fermented")
Soy sauce (Kikkoman, Yamase are naturally brewed)
Worcestershire sauce (watch for MSG and equivalents—see Rule 10)

Fresh vegetables: Highly perishable, so buy no more than 4-5 days worth of fresh vegetables at once!
Broccoli
Vine-ripened tomatoes or cherry tomatoes
Butter lettuce (other delicious lettuces: arrugula, mizuna)
Baby greens
Radish, mung bean, and all other sprouts
Radishes
Daikon radish
String beans
Snow peas
Kale (also Swiss chard. Explore the curly and colored varieties)
Corn on the cob
Carrots
Celery
Leeks
Cabbage, green or purple
Cauliflower
Green pepper
Red and yellow pepper (sweeter than green, great for salads)
Mushrooms, all types (dried mushrooms are an easier alternative due to their longer shelf life)

Dairy
Whole milk, organic, preferably unpasteurized and unhomogenized
Fresh cream
Raw milk hard cheeses (the best source is probably your local Costco. Read the ingredients and choose those listing "milk" over "pasteurized milk")
Yoghurt, plain, whole milk (all yoghurts are pasteurized)
Sour cream
Cream cheese
Cottage cheese
Butter, preferably organic and from pastured cows (will look darker yellow than from grain-fed, due to higher CLA and vitamin content)

Fruits and veggies that freeze well
Peas
Edamame soy beans (hulled or in their pods)
Shredded coconut
Coconut cream
Blueberries
Strawberries

Appendix B

Canned goods

Tomatoes, chopped without added seasoning

Sardines, smoked or not, with bones in and in olive oil or tomato sauce; no vegetable oils

Mackerel, with bones

Salmon, with bones

Smoked oysters in olive oil

Anchovies

Kippered herring

Coconut cream (frozen versions of this taste better than canned but are harder to find; check your local Asian market)

Seafood (other than canned): Check with your local fresh fish market or grocery store that sells fish on ice for fresh, seasonal catches

Oysters

Clams

Mussels

Lobster

Crab

Salmon heads (super healthy and cheap)

Fish eggs (buy no more than a few ounces, as these are highly perishable)

Dried shrimp and sardines (Oriental markets are a great source)

Meat and eggs

Organic eggs, free-range

Free-range chicken wings, legs, whole chickens, breast meat—buy with bone and skin (more flavorful)

Free-range red meat products, ground beef, New York strip, T-bone, Rib steak

Humanely raised pork products

Lamb shanks (lamb is typically pasture-raised)

"Fast foods"

Sushi

Pickled herring (look for brands with less than 8 grams of sugar per serving)

Soups and chowders from grocery store delis (check ingredients carefully; avoid vegetable oils)

Sprouted grain salads (available from Whole Foods and other health food stores)

From the deli

Roast beef

Chicken and turkey that look like sliced meat, not a sponge

Liverwurst

Smoked fish products (sold in vacuum seal near the deli)

Bubbies or other brand of fermented pickles and sauerkraut

Kimchee, fermented (best from Asian markets, ask proprietor, should have a bubbly taste)

Fermented beets (found at health food stores)

Appendix B

<u>Condiments</u>

Capers

Mustard

Roasted red peppers

Jelly (the best will have less than 10
grams of sugar per tablespoon)

Ketchup (choose a brand with the
smallest amount of sugar per
serving)

Hot chile and pepper sauces

Salsa verde

<u>Desserts</u>

Dark chocolate made with cocoa butter
or other natural fat

Ice cream made with real cream and
five or fewer other ingredients

Cookies and baked goods made using
butter or coconut oils

Jell-O (gelatin, but try cutting the sugar
by a third or more)

Appendix C

Foods to scratch off your shopping list

Not recommended:

Dried goods and pantry items

Instant oatmeal, especially flavored and sweetened

Fruity products

Fruit roll ups

Fruit drinks and punches

Jams and jellies with more than 12 grams of sugar per tablespoon

Starchy foods

Boxed cereals

Flavored crackers, and crackers made with vegetable oils or containing mono- and diglycerides

Burrito and taco shells made with corn, soy, canola, or other vegetable oil

Breads made with "wheat flour" that have a spongy texture

Breads containing mono- or di-glycerides or vegetable oils

Most pita pockets, unless sprouted and free of the above oils and additives

Snack chips, unless made with olive or other traditional oils (these will be costly)

Tater Tots and French fries

Nuts and seeds

Peanut butters or nut butters containing added sugar

Nuts or seeds roasted in vegetable oil (most say "peanut *or* vegetable oil"; peanut oil would be fine, but given the relative costs, figure on it being vegetable oil most of the time)

Candy-coated nuts and seeds, unless for dessert

Seasonings and spices

Sugar containing seasoning mixes and spice blends

"Natural flavors" (95 percent chance of containing MSG)

"Artificial flavors"

Bullion cubes

Cooking oils, sauces, and pantry items

Vegetable oils (see Rule 2 for details)

Cooking oil sprays and aerosols

Soy sauce and fish sauces containing anything "hydrolyzed"

Barbecue sauces with sugar listed more than once or as the second ingredient (see Rule 5 for other names for sugar)

Salsa with added sugar or vegetable oil

Pasta sauces with sugar in the top three ingredients, or any vegetable oil

Salad dressings (unless made with olive, sesame, or peanut oil and free of unhealthy oils)

Appendix C

Fresh vegetables
All okay!

Dairy
Non-organic dairy products
Low-fat and fat-free cheeses, yoghurts, and milk (mozzarella is an exception as "part skim" is part of the tradition)
Dips with mono- and diglycerides, or MSG, or labeled "low-fat"
Fake dairy creamers
Powdered dairy products
Cheeses containing casein
Butter substitutes, margarine, and low-cholesterol spreads
Soy milk
Rice milk

Fruits and veggies that lose nutrition rapidly while frozen
Broccoli
String beans

Canned goods
Pie fillings
Fruit cocktail and other canned fruits
Soups
Vegetables other than tomato
Boneless canned meats, i.e., tuna (compared to bone-in, these tend to be flavorless and more likely to contain MSG—a missed opportunity for bone-building minerals)
Broths and stocks (mostly salt, MSG, and artificial flavorings)
Sardines or seafood in vegetable oil

Seafood
Fish sticks and patties

Meat and eggs
Powdered eggs
Yolk-free egg products
Boneless, skinless meats (limit, see Rule 32)
Extra-lean ground beef
Extra-lean Canadian bacon
Turkey bacon
Bacon bits

Fast foods
Franchise chains

From the deli
Sandwich meats containing nitrates or nitrites
Fat-free turkey or chicken slices

Condiments
Mayo (made of olive oil is okay)
Sweet relishes
Sweet ketchups

Other products to avoid
Most frozen meals
Frozen waffles
Hot Pockets
Irradiated foods
Protein powders and drinks
Energy bars and other food bars
Foods ending in "able" such as lunchable, snackable

One Week of Breakfasts and Lunches

(Single servings unless otherwise noted)

Yoghurt Berry-Nut Parfait #1

1/2 C organic, plain, whole milk yoghurt

1/2 C of a combination of: granola made with coconut oil, raisins, dried cranberries and/or cherries, raw pumpkin seeds, cashews

Yoghurt Berry-Nut Parfait #2

1/2 C organic, plain, whole milk yoghurt

3 Tbsp raw walnuts (omega-3 fats)

3 dried apricots, diced (or cut with cooking shears)

Best-for-You Bacon and Eggs

Poached egg and 1 slice sprouted grain toast with 1-1.5 Tbsp organic butter with 2 slices nitrate-free bacon

Buttery Egg and Cheese Melt

1 pastured egg fried sunny side up in 1.5-2 Tbsp organic butter, topped with 1/8 inch thick layer of cheddar applied long enough before egg is finished cooking to melt cheese and leave yolk with a soft, moist center

German Sour-Cracker Torte

Liverwurst and hot mustard on toasted, quartered pumpernickel bread

Irish Sushi

Pickled herring pieces with freshly peeled, whole carrot on the side

Orange Ocean on Toast

Sprouted whole grain toast with generous coating of organic butter heaped with fish roe

Balsamic Tomato Bruschetta

Grape tomatoes sliced in halves and coated in olive oil, balsamic vinegar, and salt with diced basil piled high onto sprouted grain or sourdough bread and then lightly toasted

Fresh-Cream Milk with Cinnamon Toast

1 slice sprouted whole grain cinnamon-raisin toast with 1 Tbsp organic butter and 1 C fresh, whole milk with 1-2 Tbsp fresh cream added

Creamy Spiced Oat Groats

Bring 1 C oat groats and 3 C water to boil, simmer 30 minutes, then allow to sit overnight in fridge after cooling. To eat, reheat (0.5 to 1 C per person) with milk, cream, raisins, cinnamon, and your favorite nuts

BLT to the Max

Sprouted grain toast, homemade mayo, naturally cured bacon from free-range pork, and organic tomatoes, and lettuce

Egg Salad Sandwich and Capers

Egg salad made with 4 eggs, 1-2 Tbsp mayo (preferably homemade), 1-1.5 tsp mustard, 1-2 Tbsp capers or pickle relish. Spread half of this mixture over toasted sprouted grain bread. Serves 2

Coffee-Flavored Fresh Milk

1 C fresh milk, 1/8 C fresh cream, toddy coffee (soak 1/8 C grinds in 2/3 C cold water overnight, filter through large paper filter). Fresh dairy tastes heavenly when cows are grazing on grass (i.e. in warm weather)

Cucumber Basil Salad

Sliced grape tomatoes and cut cucumbers mixed in balsamic vinegar, salt, pickle juice, minced basil, and pine nuts

(See Rule 77 for more quick meal ideas)

One week of delicious dinners

Split Pea Sausage Soup

Split peas and carrots cooked in chicken broth with smoked sausage

Rosemary Roasted Chicken with Pan-Crisped Potato Slices

Whole, free-range chicken with butter/rosemary rubbed skin and sliced potatoes at bottom of pan absorbing the juices.

Greens: Pan-baked, butter-coated carrots, and broccoli

Homemade Pizza with Sausage and Wheat Berry Crust

Organic, unbleached white flour dough with 3/4 C fresh ground wheat berries, organic tomato-based sauce with fresh basil, oregano, and thyme, and sausage from pasture-raised pork

Greens: Giant organic butter lettuce and red romaine salad with capers, pine nuts, celery, carrots, and Italian dressing

Grass-Fed Burger with Caramelized Onion

Grass-fed burger with egg and oatmeal (for cohesion) and pan-caramelized onion, Bubbies pickle slices, fresh tomato, and lettuce

Greens: Arrugula, goat cheese, candied pecans, orange zest, and balsamic vinaigrette dressing

Fish Taco Melt with Cheese and Easy Hollandaise

Gently poached fresh haddock over corn tortilla with melted cheddar, hollandaise sauce (or homemade mayo). Top with sliced purple cabbage and fresh salsa (tomatoes, jalapeno, green onions, garlic, lime, cilantro, and salt)

Lamb Shank Chili with New Potatoes and Beans

Cubed lamb shank slow-cooked in Dutch oven with sprouted pinto, black, and kidney beans, carrots, potatoes, and savory brown stock made from grass-fed braised bones

Greens: Steamed Brussels sprouts in garlic butter

Made in United States
Orlando, FL
29 January 2022

14174234R00098